A Beginner's Guide

TO THE
Brain

Major Discoveries
That Will Change Your Life

For Elayne with gratitude and admiration.
Elaine

Elaine B. Johnson, Ph.D.

With a Foreword by Dr. Eric Chudler
Illustrations by Jana Hirst

Library of Congress Control Number: 2011943640

ISBN 978-0-9830956-1-3

PUBLISHER

The Teaching & Learning Compact

Overland Park, KS 66202

DEDICATION

To Tom and Thomas and
in memory of Elaine Larson

"I, / Beyond all limit of what else I' th' world,
Do love, prize, honour you."

Shakespeare. *The Tempest*. III. i. 71-73.

CONTENTS

Acknowledgments

A BEGINNER'S GUIDE TO THE BRAIN: MAJOR DISCOVERIES THAT Will Change Your Life is indebted to the work of many neuroscientists and psychologists, particularly Antonio Damasio, Joseph LeDoux, Michael Gazzaniga, Susan Greenfield, Patricia K. Kuhl, Michael Merzenich, Helen Neville, Jeanette Norden, Robert Sapolsky, and Jeffrey Schwartz. I am particularly grateful to Eric Chudler, research associate professor in the University of Washington's Department of Bioengineering. Dr. Chudler read and commented on the manuscript. Any errors are my fault, not his.

David A. Sousa, Robert Sylwester, and Patricia Wolfe were among the first non-neuroscientists to interpret the findings of brain research for educators. Their example suggested the need for a brain book with a slightly different slant, a book that encourages general readers, especially parents, business leaders, and educators, to reflect on the meaning of neuroscience for daily life and work. *A Beginner's Guide to the Brain: Major Discoveries That Will Change Your Life* discusses, for instance, how the brain forms a moral view; why humans require positive relationships; why the brain's reward system trumps external incentives; how the brain makes and breaks habits; what learning and remembering entail; and the power of thought alone to change the brain's physical structure. Dealing with these matters implies some fundamental questions: "Does knowledge of the brain's structure and function carry with it new responsibilities? If so, what actions and decisions does knowledge of the brain require of every human being, especially of parents, teachers and others in positions of leadership?"

For opportunities to study the application of brain research in schools, I am grateful to Jef Caelen, Guus Giesen, Jan Juttens, and Truus Römgens, whose efforts have made the study of the brain part of the curriculum in many schools in the Netherlands. My thanks also to Danielle Houtvast and her colleagues at De Duizendpoot Elementary School, the Netherlands, where young people speak knowingly of the brain's structure and function. Thomas Armstrong, President of Barstow Community College; Barbara Orr, Director of the Teaching & Learning Compact in Overland Park, Kansas; and Arlene Parisot, Educational Consultant for the Montana Commissioner of Higher Education and Board Member of the Montana Arts Council gave me many opportunities to find out how educators applied brain research in their classrooms.

Jane Seddon and Jan Gillet, the CEO's of Process Management International, Ltd., England; Anders Bröms, CEO of Samarbetande Konsulter, Sweden; and William Bellows, Associate Fellow at Pratt and Whitney Rocketdyne, California, generously enabled me to explore the connection between understanding the human brain and responsible action among business leaders. I am also grateful to Janice Molloy, Director of *Pegasus Communications* for her editorial advice on chapter four. The encouragement of Juanita Brown, co-author with David Isaacs of *Shaping Our Futures Through Conversations That Matter* (Barrett-Kohler) and co-founder of the World Café, an innovative system for conducting collaborative, large group conversations, was a steady help.

Gerald Wheeler, Cain Hoy, and Roger Tait provided essential technical assistance, meeting impossible deadlines with gracious good humor. Armando Benitez of Alondra Press commented helpfully on the manuscript, and Jana Hirst's illustrations made it possible to interpret complex descriptions. My husband and son, who leavened work with laughter, made writing this book a pleasant family affair.

Foreword

ADVANCES IN OUR UNDERSTANDING OF THE BRAIN ARE BEING made at an incredible pace with the new discoveries, therapies and innovations reported frequently in both scientific trade journals and popular magazines for the public. Still, the layperson may find it difficult to sift through this literature to obtain an understanding of how the brain functions and the meaning of a particular scientific study. Elaine Johnson, in her book, *A Beginner's Guide to the Brain: Major Discoveries that Will Change Your Life* helps with this process.

Elaine Johnson has successfully distilled contemporary neuroscientific topics into an enjoyable, readable book that will help everyone appreciate the workings of those three-pounds of gray matter in our heads.

Johnson takes you on a journey inside your brain. In her discussion of neuroplasticity, she explains how the brain is able to change itself and even holds the potential to repair itself. In her discussion about memory, Johnson describes how long-term memories are formed and how they interact with emotions. She analyzes the connection between emotion and reason, and she discusses how profoundly our relationships with others impact the brain. Johnson shows that relationships exert a powerful influence on the brain's structure and function.

One of Johnson's most compelling chapters focuses on the

underlying basis of morality. She reminds us that daily life and local culture wire the brain with ideas of right and wrong. Because these ideas are local and subjective, they require careful scrutiny. Thinking carefully about moral beliefs helps us enlarge our understanding of right and wrong.

Johnson's book concludes with suggestions for creating experiences that keep the brain in top shape and draw forth its full promise.

Always stimulating and informative, *A Beginner's Guide to the Brain: Major Discoveries that Will Change Your Life* is sure to help you understand what makes you, you.

ERIC H. CHUDLER, PH.D.
Research Associate Professor
Department of Bioengineering
University of Washington
Seattle, Washington

Preface

FOR THE PAST THREE DECADES, NEUROSCIENTISTS HAVE made stunning discoveries about how the human brain works. Many of these discoveries about the brain's architecture and operations reinforce one particular breakthrough—namely, that each of us has the power to change the brain's physical structure. Each of us is capable of changing our brain's structure, for instance, to raise IQ, control emotions, adopt moral principles, and modify attitudes. Furthermore each of us has the ability to influence the structure of someone else's brain. The discovery that our words and actions can actually alter the wiring in the brain of a friend, child, spouse, or colleague challenges us to think carefully about how we interact with others. Will we influence their brains to wire for more kindness, awareness, and tolerance? What impact will our words and behavior have on the wiring of an employee's brain or the brain of a child? These questions merit thoughtful consideration.

What happens in the brain that makes it possible for the brain of one person to participate in sculpting someone else's brain? What makes the brain so flexible that it changes its wiring? How does the brain rewire itself? How does the brain function? Why is it important to appreciate the brain? *A Beginner's Guide to the Brain: Major Discoveries That Will Change Your Life* explores such questions.

Each chapter in this book discusses features of the brain and suggests why it is important that everyone, particularly parents, business leaders, and educators, should understand these features. *Chapter 1. Understanding Plasticity: How Experience Changes the Brain* explores the brain's capacity to shape itself in response to the outside world. The brain is not rigid and unalterable. It is flexible. In other words, it has plasticity. Because of its plasticity, the brain changes its structure in response to daily life. Plasticity enables the brain to do such things as learn to speak the languages it hears, recover from stroke, overcome learning disabilities, and increase in intelligence. Those who understand that daily life changes the flexible brain's structure and, as a result, changes what the brain can do, live intentionally. They intentionally make decisions, engage in activities, and choose learning experiences meant to change their brains. They also look for opportunities to influence the wiring of others' brains. Understanding the brain's plasticity is the key to unlocking the brain's full potential.

Brain cells and regions communicate constantly. *Chapter 2. Making Connections: How Brain Cells and Regions Communicate* explains how this communication takes place. Human beings learn, feel, think, and imagine because brain cells and regions collaborate. The term "brain cell" can refer either to a nerve cell, called a "neuron," or to a glial cell, which supports the neuron. From birth to death, neurons connect, forming circuits that make possible everything the brain does. Neurons connect as a result of a process that is both electrical and chemical. A neuron fires an electrical charge. That charge releases a chemical molecule that joins neurons together. The place where they join is called the *synapse*. When neurons connect and stay joined, they change the brain's structure.

Just as tiny neurons interact, so do large brain regions. For instance, the two sides of the brain, regions known as the right and left hemispheres, act as one because they are connected. The thin layer covering the hemispheres, called the *cortex*, consists of four lobes. These lobes are also connected. Their connections make it possible to do such things as interpret sights and sounds, identify objects, locate objects in space, calculate an object's motion and speed, and process touch, pain, and pressure. Knowing how the brain communicates enables us to behave in ways that aid the brain's operations and processes.

Chapter 3. Memory and Emotion explores how human beings learn and remember. It points out that we learn and remember best when we engage the five senses, minimize stress, eliminate fear, generate positive emotions, discover meaning, use repetition, and practice. When the brain processes meaning, generates emotions, draws on the five senses, repeats, and practices, it is at the same time engaging the working memory, hippocampus, and long-term memory. The working memory, activated when something gets our attention, sends information to the hippocampus. The hippocampus, gateway to long-term memory, decides what facts, events, and skills the brain will store for the long term. The hippocampus favors information that holds meaning and carries positive emotion. Knowing how the brain learns and remembers enables us to cultivate brain-friendly strategies that deepen memory.

Chapter 4. How Relationships Forge the Brain shows that relationships forge the Self. Relationships do this in part by stimulating mirror neurons. Mirror neurons are special brain cells designated to imitate, or mirror, the feelings and actions one person observes in someone else. Mirror neurons wire to mirror what another person observes or feels. Given the power of mirror neurons to mimic what they see another doing or feeling, parents, teachers, and leaders appropriately ask: "Do I want people to mirror my attitude and actions right now? Does my behavior merit emulation?"

Relationships do more than activate mirror neurons to imitate actions and feelings. They also influence personality traits, intellectual abilities, and emotional make-up. Abusive or neglectful relationships wire the brain in ways that impair the intellect, stunt emotions, and twist personality. Loving relationships, however, wire the brain to feel secure and compassionate.

When relationships cause people to feel that they belong, their brain rewards them with a pleasurable sensation. When people feel rejected, their brain registers the pain of social distress. It registers this social pain in exactly the same two places that also register physical pain. The pain of not belonging is real. The brains of those who are in some way diminished by their peers—say, through bullying, mockery, public humiliation, or isolation—experience pain in the same places that respond to the physical pain of a broken leg. The knowledge that relationships influence the wiring in our own and someone else's brain calls for thoughtful interaction with everyone we encounter.

The brain's morality is the subject of *Chapter 5. Fashioning the Moral Brain*. At birth, the brain arrives equipped to distinguish right from wrong. Genes make this possible. Genes also equip humans to share a few universal moral principles. In addition, people learn morality from their family, friends, and local culture. Just as a specific culture wires the brain with its distinctive morality, so emotion influences morality. Often the *feeling* that a belief is right is enough to cause someone to embrace it. Those who become attached emotionally to an idea may willfully ignore evidence that discredits it. In that case, emotion defeats reason.

Moral beliefs become ingrained habits of thought that literally occupy space in the brain. Breaking the grip of habits of thought is possible because, as brain research shows, thought alone is sufficient to alter circuits holding habitual beliefs. Thought by itself can cause the brain to discard misguided beliefs.

The knowledge that thinking sculpts the brain challenges all human beings, especially parents, educators, and business leaders, to ask good questions, pay close attention, withhold judgment, and cultivate mindfulness. The power of thought to change the brain challenges us to respect hard evidence, be receptive to new possibilities, give a fair hearing to unpalatable ideas, and seek the fullest understanding possible. It asks that we strive always to think logically, honestly, and well.

Chapter 6. Shaping a Brain-Friendly Learning Environment makes specific recommendations about experiences that benefit the brain. Because experiences and even thoughts can change the structure and function of the malleable human brain, it is incumbent upon us to ask: "What experiences nurture brains? What things harm them?" Research shows that music, new languages, physical exercise, and positive relationships, among other things, benefit the developing brain. According to brain research, however, spending hours in front of computers, smart phones, and TV may undermine the brain's ability to pay attention, concentrate, and think deeply. Violent entertainment, furthermore, may wire the brain for violence, producing people with a predilection to act aggressively and harm others.

Does our environment generate experiences that help the malleable, plastic brain become thoughtful, reflective, intelligent, reasonable, compassionate and attentive? Do the experiences we offer children invite their brains to weave patterns, discover meaning, learn, remember, manage emotions, think critically, distinguish right from wrong, and love? Does our environment wire young brains to value education, read analytically, do their best, help others, and contribute to the community? Does it wire adults to look to the well-being of others as well as themselves?

The brain's remarkable powers make it possible for every human being to design his or her own brain. When human beings design their own brains, they also design the species. Will we shape human beings that regard others as equal in value to themselves? Will we sculpt human beings that prize and work to preserve Earth's richness, diversity, and incomparable beauty? The choices we make for the magnificent brain will decide our destiny.

CHAPTER 1

Understanding Plasticity: How Experience Changes the Brain

"Things do not change; we change."

Henry David Thoreau. *Walden: or Life in the Woods*. 1854.

THIS BOOK IS ABOUT HOW TO TAKE CHARGE OF YOUR BRAIN. Thirty-five years ago, it could not have been written. In those days, because of limited technology, scientists mainly studied dead or damaged brains. Such studies led them to the entrenched conviction that the blob of tissue securely lodged inside the skull was fixed at birth and nothing could be done to change it. Today, however, new technology allows scientists to study the living, healthy brain and to photograph the brain in action. In the mid 1980s, for example, Magnetic resonance imaging (MRI) was developed to show how the brain uses oxygen. When a part of the brain is busy doing something, it needs more oxygen and glucose than it needs when it is at rest. An increase in an area's oxygen and glucose signifies an increase in its activity. The MRI tracks the brain's use of oxygen by means of radio waves and powerful magnets. PET, positron emission tomography, also identifies active areas of the brain. It uses a radioactive isotope injected into the blood. When the patient does something like sing or count, the isotope makes it possible to follow the brain's use of glucose and oxygen. Thanks to MRIs and PET scans, as well as other sophisticated technology, scientists have proved beyond a doubt that the brain is not fixed, unalterable and limited by genetic inheritance. On the contrary, it changes constantly. Its ability to change is called *plasticity*.[1]

Arguably the most remarkable discovery of neuroscience in recent years, one that gives hope to all human beings, is the discovery that the brain is *plastic*. The term *plastic*, a synonym for *flexible* and *malleable*, means that the brain changes as its cells connect and reconnect in response to experience.[2] As we journey through the day, experience causes brain cells to forge new connections and terminate unsatisfactory wiring. The malleable brain is "like a living creature . . . that can grow and change."[3] Reacting to whatever we do—whether we read, drive a car, text message, play video games, jog, or laugh with friends—the dynamic brain forges new connections. A self-organizing, living system, it revises and reorganizes the size of its neurons, the size of its regions, the strength of its wiring, and its functions[4] until the day we die. From basic facts about the brain to how we learn language, increase IQ, and overcome brain damage, this chapter shows readers what plasticity means for them.

Brain Basics

Small enough to be balanced in the palm of one hand, composed of white, cream, and pink colors, the average adult brain has the consistency of cottage cheese, cooked oatmeal, or soft butter. Soft and fragile, it needs protection. Shaking an infant, riding a bike without wearing a helmet, or, some contend, head butting a soccer ball, put the fragile brain at risk.

The average adult male brain weighs about 1400 grams, or 3.09 pounds. The average adult female brain, slightly smaller, weighs about 1300 grams, or 2.87 pounds.[5] This discrepancy, which may tempt a woman to infer that she can do more with less, occurs because the brain is proportioned to the size of the body, and women's bodies are generally smaller than men's.[6]

The brain achieves its adult weight very quickly. By age two, a child's brain reaches three-quarters of its adult weight. By age four or five, the child's brain reaches 90 to 95 percent of its adult weight. Between the ages of 14 and 16, the typical brain achieves its full adult weight of approximately three pounds. This rapid increase in size happens because daily life causes brain cells—neurons—to connect. Experience configures the plastic brain.

Once the brain reaches its adult weight of three pounds, it is not yet finished. Its architecture—the elegant arrangement of neurons into columns, clusters, and layers—is not fully organized until a person's late twenties. The prefrontal cortex also remains incomplete until the late twenties.[7] Because our words, thoughts, and actions help design the prefrontal cortex, because the brain's plasticity allows us to influence it, it is important that we understand the significant role the prefrontal cortex plays.

The prefrontal cortex

Located just behind the forehead, the prefrontal cortex does more than any other region of the brain to make us human. It gives us our unique sense of self, our mind, the personality we designate with the pronoun "I." In addition, it acts as the brain's CEO.[8] As the brain's primary executive area, the prefrontal cortex makes it possible to set a goal, figure out steps leading to that goal, evaluate successes and failures along the way, recognize the implications of actions, and anticipate consequences.

In addition, the prefrontal cortex enables us to speculate about abstractions such as justice and goodness, and it equips us to maneuver in the concrete world that requires attending to minute details and distinguishing between the trivial and significant.

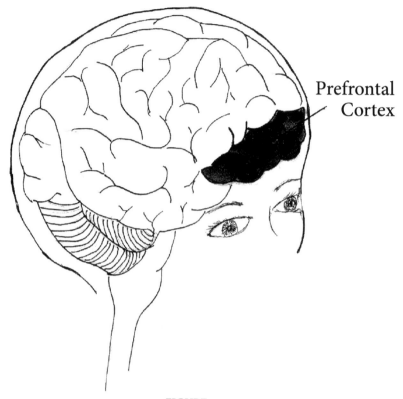

Prefrontal
Cortex

FIGURE 1

As we navigate through the day, meeting deadlines, assessing information, facing moral choices, and socializing with friends, we rely on the prefrontal cortex for more than the ability to identify specific details, theorize, prioritize, and plan ahead. We also rely on it to make sense of emotion. Connected to the amygdala, the brain's emotional center, the prefrontal cortex lets us reason about emotion, regulate the intensity of our emotions, control impulses, and adjust to another's emotions.[9] Given its many critical functions, it is easy to see that the prefrontal cortex, which "endows the world with meaning and our lives with a sense of purpose,"[10] warrants careful nurturing. What we do each day wires and rewires it.

The effects of a damaged prefrontal cortex: the story of Phineas Gage

The role of the prefrontal cortex in controlling emotions and governing sophisticated mental operations is illustrated by the famous nineteenth-century case of Phineas Gage. Gage was a highly respected, self-disciplined, emotionally stable railroad foreman. At 26, he was the popular leader of a gang of men who dynamited granite in Vermont to clear the way for new railroad track. The dynamiters always followed a set routine. First the men put coarse-grained gunpowder into a small hole. After placing a long fuse in the powder, they filled the rest of the hole with sand. Finally Gage tamped down the sand with his three foot, seven inch long, thirteen and a half pound tamping iron. Then he shouted a warning, lit the fuse, and ran.

On September 13, 1848, someone neglected to put sand on top of the gunpowder. This mistake meant that when Gage bent over his tamping iron to tap the sand, he hit not sand, but exposed gunpowder and granite. When the tamping iron struck granite, it ignited a spark. The spark hit the exposed powder, causing a massive explosion. The explosion blew the tamping iron through Phineas Gage's left cheekbone, up behind Gage's left eye, through the front of his brain, and out the middle of his forehead near the hairline. The iron landed about thirty feet away, covered with blood and brain. Gage should have died from this blow to the prefrontal cortex, but amazingly he was awake and talkative after the accident. Two days later, he did develop a dangerous fever and infection, but by the end of ten weeks, Gage's body had fully recovered. His mind, however, did not recover.

According to his physician, John Martyn Harlow, Gage became unreliable, indecisive, "fitful, irreverent, indulging at times in the grossest profanity (which was not previously his custom) manifesting but little deference for his fellows, impatient of restraint or advice when it conflicts with his desires . . . A child in his intellectual capacities and manifestations, he has the animal passions of a strong man."[11] With the decimation of his prefrontal cortex, Gage lost his social judgment, inhibitions, initiative, foresight, and logical capacities. Moving from place to place and job to job, he could never find contentment and peace. He died of a seizure on May 21, 1860. Phineas Gage's experience clarifies the role of the prefrontal cortex. The prefrontal cortex brings together in one place attention, thinking, memory, and emotion, defines the "I," and harbors conscience.

The slow development of this critical brain area raises an interesting ethical question. If a fifteen-year old commits a crime, does his immature prefrontal cortex excuse criminal behavior? Can he say, "My brain made me do it?" The Supreme Court in a landmark case struck down the death penalty for murderers under the age of eighteen partly on the grounds that the prefrontal cortex of adolescents is not complete until the late twenties.[12] Whatever one's ethical position, it is clear that the gradual development of the prefrontal cortex implies the need for adults to be an adolescent's prefrontal cortex.

Plasticity and Growth

Although the prefrontal cortex develops gradually, in general the young brain grows with phenomenal speed. The question is, "What causes this growth?" The short answer is "Plasticity." Growth does not occur because the young brain is acquiring more *neurons*. The term *neuron* refers to one of two kinds of brain cell. The other kind, *glial cells*, lends support to neurons. Neurons are the brain cells that allow us to do everything humans do—to think, feel, move, breathe and carry on life. At birth the brain comes equipped with virtually its entire allotment of one hundred billion neurons.[13] These are the neurons it uses throughout life.

Recently scientists were astonished to find that some new neurons actually do emerge very gradually in a few areas of the adult brain. Although little is understood about this new cell growth—neurogenesis—it is certain that it does not cause the brain's growth during childhood and adolescence. The young brain grows because its billions of neurons connect with one other.

Neurons connect in response to the surrounding environment, the outside world that reaches neurons through movement and the five senses. We touch, taste, see, hear, feel, and move through each day. Movement and the five senses relay signals to the brain. When these signals—nerve impulses—reach the brain, they cause neurons to connect with one another, forming circuits. The formation of new circuits causes the brain to change and grow.[14] The connections that neurons make depend on environment. "Any small change in the . . . lifestyle or environment," as scientist Susan Greenfield notes, "will be reflected in a change in neuronal circuitry.... It is connections that are important. . . ."[15] Every time you dine with a friend, brush snow off a windshield, or see a new movie, neurons connect. If you go for a walk, that walk sends signals to the brain that result in neural connections. As the day's events and activities cause neurons to connect, these connections alter the brain's physical architecture. Because specific experiences shape each brain, even the brains of identical twins differ from one another.[16]

Genes and environment collaborate

It is indeed a very good thing that the brain is plastic because at birth it arrives with considerable assembly required. Genes dispose brain cells—prepare brain cells—to connect properly, but innumerable connections remain to be made only after the baby is born. Genes provide the blueprint for these connections. They are like the frame of the house. Environment, however, completes the brain. It supplies everything that goes into that house.[17] The power of environment to shape the brain is illustrated by the development of our ability to hear, speak, and see.[18]

Hearing, speaking, seeing

A mature fetus can hear its mother's voice. However, the system that hears, involving mainly the auditory cortex, is incomplete at birth. It matures over time and in response to experience.[19] The more sounds one hears, the more circuits the brain forms. Children who consistently hear a wide variety of sounds, such as leaves blowing in the wind, crashing waves, violin music, and nursery rhymes develop auditory circuits that let them, as adults, detect subtle speech patterns and musical nuances. When a sound is not heard, the neurons that our genes provided to receive that sound atrophy.[20]

The effect of sound on neurons is illustrated by the way children learn their native language. From birth, a child possesses the ability to recognize the individual sounds (phonemes) of every one of the six thousand languages spoken on earth. All babies come genetically equipped to hear every single sound. Genes designate particular brain cells in the baby's brain—neurons located in the auditory cortex—to receive particular sounds. If the specific neurons designated to handle an exact sound do not receive that sound, then those neurons will die. For example, if the brain never hears the "th" sound, then the neurons genetically assigned to receive the "th" sound will atrophy.

The more the infant hears a single sound, such as "th", the more that "th" is wired into a tiny cluster of neural circuits in the brain's auditory cortex. The cluster of neurons holding "th" comes alive with electrical activity when—and *only* when—that distinctive "th" sound enters the child's ear and passes to the brain. Circuits of neurons in your brain hold all the sounds of your native language; the sounds of the language you speak are embedded in neurons in your brain. Experience decides what languages your brain hears and acquires. Experience decides if Norwegian sounds like gibberish to you or carries meaning.

An infant's brain is able only for a short time to encode every new sound that comes its way. Quickly its auditory cortex loses the ability to wire neurons to hold particular sounds. To retain particular sounds, an infant must hear them when it is between six months and ten months old. For instance, at seven months, Japanese babies easily distinguish the sound of an English "r" from the sound of an English "l." By nine months, however, the door to language begins slowly to swing shut. At ten months, Japanese-speaking babies are deaf to the difference between "r" and "l." Because their local language did not contain "l," the neurons genetically designated to distinguish "l" withered and died. Unfamiliar languages sound like noise because the brain has not put the sounds of that unfamiliar language into circuits.[21] They are not embedded in the brain.

Having acquired sounds, the baby's brain achieves the remarkable feat of formulating words, grasping their meaning, learning rules of grammar, and mastering word order. They understand that word order alone gives "The ball hit Fred" a different meaning from "Fred hit the ball."

Personal social interaction involving one-on-one conversations, eye contact, gesturing, and facial expressions all teach children sounds and words far more effectively than does the virtual world of computer and television screens.[22] By the age of three, typically children have learned about one thousand words.

Interestingly, research at the University of Chicago shows that if parents talk to a two-year old frequently, they will increase the size of that child's vocabulary for the rest of his or her life.[23]

Vision

Experience decides not only the language children speak and the range of their vocabulary, but also it affects their vision. Visual experiences cause neurons in the visual cortex to connect and become strong. Unused, these neurons shrivel and disappear. Immediately after birth, visual acuity is only about a twentieth of what it will be by the age of five. An environment that provides a child with bright colors, a variety of bold geometric shapes, and new things to look at promotes the development of visual acuity.[24] If for some reason a child's eye does not receive signals from the outside world, however, vision will not develop properly.

The misfortune of an Italian infant illustrates the brain's dependence on experience. Parents noticed that their infant had contracted a mild eye infection. Long before brain science had discovered that signals from the outside world trigger neurons to connect in the visual system, the doctor treated the infection with medicine and then covered the eye for two weeks with a bandage. At the end of two weeks, the doctor removed the bandage. The infection was gone, but the eye remained forever blind. It was blind because the bandage kept signals from the outside world from reaching the neurons genetically appointed to serve the bandaged eye. When the neurons attached to the bandaged eye received no signals, they could not establish the eye-to-brain circuits required for vision.[25] Concluding that the bandaged eye did not need the neurons meant to serve it, the brain allowed neurons from the good eye to take over all connections to the visual cortex.

Today, of course, physicians are mindful that the brain has

plasticity. They realize that if an infant's cataract is not removed early, that cataract will prevent the brain from receiving messages from the senses. Deprived of sensory signals, neurons meant to serve the cataract eye would fail to establish necessary circuitry, resulting in blindness.

The Italian infant's experience amounts to a cautionary tale. It underscores the point that to thrive, neurons require stimulation from the outside world. Deprived of stimulation, neglected neurons will seek other neural relationships, or they will perish.[26]

Rewiring Regions

Stimulation from the outside world does far more, of course, than influence the development of vision and hearing. Signals from the environment can also transform the function of entire brain regions. Genes designate specific regions in the brain to do specific tasks. However, the environment can compel these regions to perform a task that genes did not intend.[27] The life someone leads can actually change the operation of a brain region. The experiments of Alvara Pascual-Leone and Norihiro Sadato, building on Mike Merzenich's ground-breaking work on plasticity, prove that a brain region intended to process information from one sense can be recruited to process information from a different sense.

The job of the visual cortex in the occipital lobe, for example, is to process vision. The function of this visual region can be changed, however, to process touch.[28] The eyes of a blind person do not transmit signals to the visual cortex. In the past, working without the aid of modern technology, scientists concluded that a blind person's visual cortex sat abandoned and wasted. Today we know that the visual cortex does not sit empty and unused. Rather than waste this big expanse of territory, the brain converts it to new purposes. Blind children who learn to use Braille before they are fifteen years old rely so much on their fingers that they transmit the sensation of touch not only to the somatosensory cortex, the area that always deals with touch, but also to the visual cortex. Signals from the fingers cause touch circuits to take up squatter's rights in the visual cortex. These touch circuits change the visual cortex from a region that handles sight to a region that processes the sense of touch.

Just as blind children who use Braille are able to rezone the seemingly superfluous visual cortex to handle touch, so deaf children are able to re-zone the auditory cortex to aid vision. Although the auditory cortex of a deaf child does not process sound, this region does not go unused. Visual signals remake the auditory cortex to enhance peripheral vision.[29]

Any region in the cortex of the malleable brain is capable of changing its function to process whatever signals reach it. This adjustment is possible because all signals from the five senses become electrical patterns once they reach the brain. Electrical patterns are the universal language of the brain. Consequently every region understands and can process them.[30]

The malleable brain's capacity to process signals, refashioning the brain's structure and function, offers great hope to those afflicted with missing or damaged neurons.[31]

Constraint Theory

Until recently, the help offered to people suffering from damaged or missing neurons reflected the conviction that when brain cells died, or failed to develop properly, the brain lost forever the functions that those cells performed. This belief in a fixed, unalterable brain led to the popularity of *compensation therapy*. Compensation therapy recommends working around a problem. If a man finds reading difficult, provide him with audiotapes. If a woman is slow filling out forms or taking tests, give her more time. If a college student cannot follow the logic in a philosopher's argument, give the student an outline that color codes the argument's main points. Use compensations, in other words, to circumvent the brain's deficiency.[32]

Compensation therapy seemed an excellent help until neuroscientists discovered that[33] neurons "connect, separate, and form new relationships with other neurons,"[34] that they do so throughout one's life, and that they wire in response to very precise activities.[35] These discoveries about the malleable brain have produced *constraint therapy,* a method for retrieving lost brain functions. Unlike compensation therapy, which does not rewire the brain, constraint therapy seeks to re-configure neurons, in that way retrieving the brain's lost functions.

Edward Taub, working at the Taub Clinic of the University of Alabama, originated constraint therapy. Constraint therapy is based on the new understanding that because of the brain's plasticity, good cells can take over the work of injured cells. The question is, "How can one make that happen?" What strategies force the brain's good cells to substitute for damaged cells? Taub and his colleagues at the Taub Clinic treated a stroke victim whose right arm hung limp at his side by binding the patient's good left arm in a sling. Because his good left arm was immobilized, the patient had no alternative but to use the damaged right arm. Forced to use the injured limb for hours each day doing ordinary household chores and activities, the stroke patient eventually generated good neurons to take control of that limb, and it recovered.

This experience illustrates the principle of constraint theory. Constantly making the afflicted area work hard galvanizes healthy neurons into replacing injured or missing brain cells. In time, the replacement cells reclaim lost ability. The importance of sustained hard work is evident in the case of the patient who lost her ability to pronounce words as a result of a stroke. Unable to formulate clear words, the patient at first compensated by drawing pictures and using gestures to convey meaning. Taub required her to abandon these compensations and instead to rely again and again on certain basic language rules. The many hours and weeks the patient spent applying these rules gradually rewired her brain to let her speak again.

Taub's clinic discovered that "training is more effective if the skill relates to everyday life."[36] Training that makes sense, that has meaning because it connects to the real world, helps patients recover.

Constraint theory does more than encourage physicians to devise strategies that re-configure the brain. It also suggests that parents and educators may be able to help children surmount certain learning difficulties. Asking a child to accomplish a difficult task rather than avoid it may well give that child a chance to strengthen his or her brain. A child's poor handwriting, for instance, may originate from both a weak visual memory and a failure of muscle coordination. To address these problems, constraint therapy might ask the child to trace intricate Chinese or Russian letters or other complex lines. Tracing these unfamiliar letters and lines strengthens the visual memory by stimulating visual neurons. Tracing also strengthens muscle control by stimulating motor neurons.

A child who cannot remember even brief oral directions or messages may lack neurons that affect the auditory memory. To strengthen the auditory memory, constraint therapy might ask that child to learn and recite long poems, especially long poems in foreign languages. It might ask her to listen carefully to several brief paragraphs and immediately repeat exactly what she heard.[37]

Another kind of constraint therapy addresses the problem of dyslexia. People with dyslexia confuse letters and sounds. Research by neuroscientist Michael Merzenich indicates that dyslexia results not from vision problems, but from hearing problems. If missing or damaged circuitry in the auditory cortex does not let us hear the difference between so-called "fast" sounds like b, d, and p, then we will find it hard to distinguish between "day," "pay" and "bay." If we cannot hear the difference between the "d" in "day," the "p" in pay, and the "b" in "bay," then we cannot blend these consonant sounds with other sounds (phonemes). If we are unable to recognize these sounds, we will find it difficult to read, which depends on matching letters to sounds.

Drawing on principles of constraint therapy, Michael Merzenich and his colleagues created software called *Fast ForWord*. This software plays "fast" sounds—b, p, d—at an extremely slow pace. When these sounds are played very slowly, dyslexic children can distinguish among them. If children often hear these sounds played very slowly, their malleable brains form new auditory circuits to hold these sounds. Success takes work. To experience changes in the brain's circuits, children practice for about ninety minutes a day, five days a week, for at least eight weeks. This sustained practice wires the brain with new circuits that replace the problem neurons. The newly configured neurons permit children to hear the "fast" sounds at a normal rate and, as a result, read them.[38]

I.Q.

Just as the brain's plasticity enables the brain to regain lost functions, so plasticity enables neurons to communicate in ways that increase IQ. For centuries, popular wisdom regarded intelligence as absolutely fixed. Neuroscientists are concluding, however, that experience can raise or lower IQ by as much as twenty points.[39] The way we use our brain sharpens or limits our intelligence.

The old view of IQ holds that intelligence is one thing, a single, measurable entity, like a single cup. Furthermore, from the day we are born, intelligence is unalterable. Limited forever by genetic inheritance, nothing can be done to increase or diminish it. Intelligence is like a cup built to hold eight, and only eight, ounces.

This narrow idea of intelligence has been challenged and is being supplanted by a radical new understanding. Intelligence is not a single thing, and it is not fixed at birth. On the contrary, it is malleable—it can increase or diminish, and it is multiple—it comes in many forms.

The claim that everyone has many kinds of intelligence, not one single kind, originated with Harvard psychology professor Howard Gardner. Gardner says in *Frames of Mind: the Theory of Multiple Intelligences* (1983), "There is persuasive evidence for the existence of several autonomous human. . . intelligences . . . [that are] relatively independent of one another . . ."[40] Although many dispute Gardner's findings,[41] psychologist Richard E. Nisbett agrees with Gardner that neurological evidence supports identifying different forms of intelligence with specific areas of the brain.[42] A number of relatively independent systems seems to constitute multiple intelligences.[43] Gardner identifies these intelligences as linguistic, musical, logical-mathematical, spatial, bodily-kinesthetic, interpersonal, intrapersonal, and existentialist. The wiring for these intelligences is configured differently in every brain, and these distinctive configurations change as we live daily life. Life alters intelligence.

The fact that intelligence grows or diminishes as a result of experience has stunning implications. As Richard E. Nisbett observes in *Intelligence and How to Get It,* IQ, whether intelligence is going to be high or low "very much depends on environmental factors that have nothing to do with genes. . . .Being

"Intelligence grows or diminishes as a result of experience."

raised under conditions highly favorable to intelligence has a huge effect on IQ."[44] *There are no bad genes, just bad environments.*

Intelligence, affected as it is by experience, cannot be measured or even understood in social and physical isolation from the world. No longer do scientists believe, as theoretical neurophysiologist William Calvin points out, that intelligence can be reduced to a "simple number on a rating scale." An IQ number merely signifies the results of tests of verbal comprehension, mathematical fluency, and inductive and deductive reasoning. Such a number excludes the reality that "intelligence is a process . . . It's about improvisation. . . It's a way, involving many brain regions, by which we grope for new meanings."[45] If the world offers children a nurturing environment, their intelligence will grow. Children do not know what powers reside within them until daily life draws forth their promise.

Neuroscience professor Helen Neville's experiment with a Head Start program illustrates the power of environment to raise IQ. Neville set up an experiment involving two hundred Head Start children. These children, all from families at or below the poverty level, ranged in age from three to five-years. Before Neville intervened, they had been divided into groups of eighteen. Each group of eighteen children met daily with one, or, at the most, two teachers. Neville divided the children into groups of five and assigned one teacher to each group. Five children and their teacher met forty minutes a day every day for eight weeks. During this time, the children worked specifically on paying attention, visual and spatial skills, and language. After just eight weeks, their language, memory, and number skills had improved significantly. Furthermore, their IQs had increased.[46] Neville's experiment demonstrates that the success of children depends on the opportunities adults give them.

We human beings are born genetically endowed with malleable, plastic brains designed to be powerful, intelligent, and resilient.

Because of its plasticity, the brain wires and rewires, altering its physical structure. Plasticity helps the brain think abstractly, solve practical problems, plan ahead, and work hard to attain goals. Plasticity enables healthy brain cells to replace irreversibly damaged neurons, returning both brain and body to health. Plasticity permits us to draw on each day's opportunities to raise our IQ. How many people intentionally take advantage of the brain's plasticity? Will you?

Precisely what happens when infinitesimally small neurons invisible to the naked eye connect, and what happens when large regions cooperate is the subject of the next chapter. Awareness of these processes encourages us to take charge of our malleable brain. It helps us unleash the brain's full potential.

Endnotes: Chapter 1

1. Susan A. Greenfield, *The Human Brain: A Guided Tour* (New York: Basic Books, 1997), pp. 82; 3, 5, 27-30, 73. The CAT scan, computerized axial tomography ("tomo" comes from "tomos," the Greek word for "section"), in use since the early 1970s, causes an X-ray beam to move completely around a patient's head, generating visual "slices" of the entire brain and sending images to a screen. In this way, it captures abnormalities such as tumors or tissue loss. See also Rita Carter, *Mapping the Mind* (Berkeley: University of California Press, 1998), p. 13; Richard Restak, *The Secret Life of the Brain* (New York: The Dana Press and Joseph Henry Press, 2001), p. xviii; Greenfield, pp. 27-30; Greenfield, p. 28: "Positrons are fundamental particles similar to electrons except that they have a positive charge. Radioactive oxygen atoms incorporated into either glucose or water molecules are injected intravenously. The radioactive label is then carried by the blood into the brain. The emitted positrons collide with electrons in other molecules within the brain and mutually annihilate each other. The burst of energy that results forms a gamma ray that is of sufficiently high energy to penetrate through the skull and be detected outside of the head. . . .With PET, it is possible to show different active areas according to tasks as subtly different as saying words compared with reading words." A drawback of PET is that it requires noting the precise instant when the radioactive solution reaches the brain. See also on new technology Richard Restak, pp. xviii-xx; Robert Sylwester, *A Celebration of Neurons: An Educator's Guide to the Human Brain* (Alexandria, VA: Association for Supervision and Curriculum Development, 1995), pp. 13-14. The electron microscope, which shows molecules in brain cells, is another technological advance that aids brain research.

2. Daniel J. Siegel, *The Mindful Brain* (W. W. Norton & Co., 2007), p. 96.

3. Michael Merzenich, cited by Norman Doidge, *The Brain That Changes Itself* (New York: Viking, 2007), p. 47.

4. On the plastic brain's response to environment, see Gerald Edelman, *Second Nature: Brain Science and Human Knowledge* (New Haven: Yale University Press), p. 41; Sharon Begley, "How the Brain Rewires Itself," *Time* (January 29, 2007), p. 74; Richard Restak, p. xiii; Michael Merzenich, "Plasticity and the Brain," OHSU Brain Awareness Lecture Series, January 26, 2009; Elkhonon Goldberg, *The Executive Brain* (London: Oxford University Press, 2001), pp. 23-29.

5. Various textbooks cite these figures. See for confirmation <http://faculty.Washington. edu/chudler/facts.html>. However, Michael S. Sweeney says in *Brain: The Complete Mind* (Washington D. C.: National Geographic, 2009), p. 37, that the average adult male brain weighs 3.5 pounds, and the average adult female brain weighs 3.2 pounds. His figures are unusually high.

6. Although this book does not compare male and female brains, new studies do reveal intriguing similarities and differences. See, for example, Louann Brizendine, *The Female Brain* (New York: Broadway Books, 2006), pp. 4-6,174-75,123-31; Lori Oliwenstein, "The Most Important Sex Organ," in *Your Brain: A User's Guide* (New York: Time Inc., 2009), pp. 33-36; Antonio Damasio, *Descartes' Error: Emotion, Reason, and the Human Brain* (New York: Avon Books, 1994), pp. 987-88: "The brain and the body are indissociably integrated . . . . There are two principle routes of interconnection. The route usually thought of first is made of sensory and motor peripheral nerves which carry signals from every part of the body to the brain, and from the brain to every part of the body. The other route . . . is the bloodstream; it carries chemical signals such as hormones, neurotransmitters, and modulators. . . . Consider that the brain receives signals not only from the body but, in some of its sectors, from parts of itself that receive signals from the body!"

7. Megan Gunnar, "The Impact of Early Adversity on Brain Development: How the Brain

Recovers from Stress," lecture delivered in Portland, Oregon, at the Oregon Conference on Early Childhood, May 1, 2009. Professor Gunnar emphasizes that early experiences influence the brain's architecture and function. By age five, according to Gunnar, 90% of the brain's mass is developed. Others think that the child's brain is 90 to 95 percent of its adult size by the age of six. See, e.g., Alice Park, "What Makes Teens Tick," *Time* (May 10, 2004,) p. 59. Dr. Jay Giedd, chief of brain imaging at NIMH, says that the brain develops from back to front, so that regions receiving sensory signals and controlling vision, hearing, touch, and spatial processing develop earliest. Giedd is cited in Park, p. 59.

8. Louis Cozolino, *The Neuroscience of Human Relationships* (New York: W.W. Norton & Company, 2006), p. 53.

9. Elkhonon Goldberg, *The Executive Brain: Frontal Lobes and the Civilized Mind*. Oxford: Oxford University Press, 2001), p. 36; Restak, p. 76; Greenfield, *Human Brain,* 19-20. Cozolino, pp. 54, 277-278. The prefrontal cortex, a large area of the frontal cortex is located in front of— anterior to—the primary cortex and the secondary motor cortex. For information on its role, see Cozolino, pp. 276ff. According to Ekhonon Goldberg, pp. 36-37, "the prefrontal cortex is . . . directly interconnected with every distinct functional unit of the brain" including "the premotor cortex, basal ganglia, and the cerebellum, all involved in various aspects of motor control and movements.. . .Only the prefrontal cortex is embedded in such a richly networked pattern of neural pathways. This unique connectivity makes the frontal lobes singularly suited for coordinating and integrating the work of all the other brain structures . . . ." pp. 36-37.

10. Carter, p. 182.

11. John Fleischman, *Phineas Gage: A Gruesome but True Story about Brain Science* (Boston: Houghton Mifflin Company, 2002), p. 22. See also pp. 1-21.

12. For the Supreme Court case on this issue, see "Roper v. Simmons," (No. 03-633) 543 U.S. 551 (2005); see also Jeffrey Rosen, "The Brain on the Stand," *The New* York Times, March 11, 2007, <http://www.nytimes.com/preview20;07/03/11/magazine> downloaded 9/16/10.

13. Sweeney, p. 16. "Except for the hippocampus and the olfactory bulb, where new neurons have been shown to grow from stem cells, the neurons a person has at birth are all he or she will ever have." Neurogenesis occurs in two places in the adult brain—the olfactory bulb and the dentate gyrus, a subsystem of the hippocampus. Elizabeth Gould and Charles Gross of Princeton established that neurogenesis occurs in the dentate gyrus of the adult brain's hippocampus. See also Sue Halpern, "Forgetting is the New Normal," *Your Brain: A User's Guide,* ed. Jeffrey Kluger (New York: Time Books, Time Inc, 2009), pp. 72-76. Halpern notes that the brain produces neurons throughout life in the olfactory bulb and the dentate gyrus of the hippocampus. p. 74.

14. Greenfield, pp. 33-34, 54, 116.

15. Greenfield, pp. 115-119.

16. Edelman, p. 22.

17. Megan Gunnar said in her lecture given on May 1, 2009, at the OHSU Conference on Early Childhood in Portland, Oregon, that there are windows of opportunity—sensitive periods—for brain development. These sensitive periods are responsive to in-put from the environment. Environment activates the senses, and the senses then send signals to the brain that trigger connections among neurons. When neurons connect to form circuits, these circuits generate development of skills. Developing skills at one level makes it possible to grow neurons that equip the brain to acquire skills at the next level. Development is cumulative.

18. For insights into early language and brain development, the work of Dr. Patricia K. Kuhl, Co-Director of the University of Washington Institute for Learning & Brain Sciences, is particularly helpful. See, e.g., Patricia Kuhl and Maritza Rivera-Gaxiola, "Neural Substrates of Language Acquisition," *Annual Review of Neuroscience,* 2008, 31:511-34 <neuro. annualreviews.org. 2008> ; Alison Gopnik, Andrew Meltzoff, Patricia K. Kuhl, *Scientists in the Crib: What Early Learning Tells Us About the Mind*(New York: Harper, 2001).

19. Daniel J. Levitin, *This is Your Brain on Music* (New York: Plume, 2007), pp. 1-27; 109-120.

20. Sylwester, pp. 20-21.

21. See Jeanette Norden, *Understanding the Brain* (Cantilly, Virginia: The Teaching Company, 2007), pp. 85-91, 104-107. Norden is Professor of Cell and Developmental Biology in the School of Medicine and Professor of Neurosciences in the College of Arts and Sciences at Vanderbilt University. See also Jeffrey Kluger, "Language and the Baby Brain," *Your Brain: A User's Guide,*" (New York: Time Inc., 2009), p. 26: Kluger explains that a baby's brain learns languages easily in part because its individual neurons "connect to as many as 15,000 other neurons, and each of those 15,000 then branch out in 15,000 other ways...Adult brains have about a third fewer links per neuron."

22. Dr. Patricia Kuhl's book *The Scientist in the Crib* speaks to this issue, as does her article appearing in the *Daily Herald* (3 August 2009).

23. John Ratey, *A User's Guide to the Brain* (New York: Vintage, 2002), p. 41.

24. Sylwester, pp. 20, 61-62.

25. Greenfield, p. 114.

26. Greenfield, pp. 113-114.

27. Sharon Begley, "How the Brain Rewires Itself," *Time* (29 Jan. 2007), p. 74.

28. Begley, "How the Brain Rewires Itself," p. 74.

29. Sharon Begley, *Train Your Mind, Change Your Brain* (New York: Ballantine Books, 2007), pp. 79-101.

30. Begley, *Train Your Mind,* pp. 58-104, 129-130.

31. Begley, "How the Brain Rewires Itself," p. 74.

32. Norman Doidge, *The Brain that Changes Itself* (New York: Viking, 2007), pp. xiii-xiv.

33. Greenfield, pp. 23-24; 27. Michael Merzenich observed in a lecture presented on January 26, 2010, as part of the OHSU Brain Awareness Lecture Series, that the brain modifies itself continuously as it acquires information and new skills.

34. Sweeney, *Brain: The Complete Mind,* p. 13.

35. Steven Hyman, "Susceptibility and 'Second Hits,'" in *States of Mind: New Discoveries about How our Brains Make Us Who We Are,* ed. Roberta Conlan (New York: Wiley, 1999), pp. 9-28.

36. Doidge, pp. 153-155.

37. Doidge, pp. 153-159.

38. On constraint theory and the work of Michael Merzenich, see Doidge, pp. 68-87; 32-43. Research indictes that because singing uses a different area of the brain than is involved in speech, one form of constraint therapy for stroke victims who have lost the capacity to speak, having damaged the left side of the brain, involves asking them to sing. Singing seems to build circuits that enable them to speak. At first, the right side, the singing centre, has trouble fulfilling the role of speech. But as patients practice putting their words to simple songs, they regain the ability to form intelligible words. On this see Victoria Gill, science reporter, "Singing 'rewires' damaged brain," *BBC News* <http://newsvote.bbc.co.uk/mpapps/pagetoos > June 24, 2010.

39. Doidge, p. 209. Doidge cites Prof. Pascual-Leone's use of the metaphor equating the snow-covered hill with genetic inheritance and tracks in the snow with brain circuits developed through experience. According to The National Academy of Sciences, experience can raise or lower IQ by as much as twenty points.

40. Howard Gardner. *Frames of Mind: The Theory of Multiple Intelligences* (New York: Basic Books, 1983), pp. 8-9.

41. For critiques of Gardner's theory of multiple intelligences see, for example, Nathan Brody. *Intelligence.* 2nd ed. (New York: Academic Press, 1992); R. J. Sternberg. *The Triarchic Mind: A New Theory of Human Intelligence* (New York: Penguin Books, 1988). See also "Some Critiques of Howard Earl Gardner's Multiple Intelligences Theory," <http://www.igs.net/~cmorris/critiques.html>

42. Richard E. Nisbett, *Intelligence and How to Get It* (New York: W. W. Norton & Company, 2009), p. 14.

43. Gardner, p. 9.

44. Nisbett, pp. 2, 32; Robert J. Sternberg says in *Successful Intelligence* (New York: Plume Book, 1997), p. 49, that intelligence is the ability to act differently in different social contexts. It is the ability to "capitalize on . . . strengths and . . . remedy . . . weaknesses."

45. William H. Calvin, *How Brains Think: Evolving Intelligence Then and Now* (New York: Basic Books, 1996), pp. 2, 10-11.

46. Helen Neville, described the Head Start experiment in her lecture, "Effects of Environment on the Brain," given on May 1, 2009, in Portland, Oregon at the Oregon Conference on Early Childhood. For further information, see the DVD "Changing Brains: Effects of Experience on Human Brain Development" produced by Neville and her colleagues at the University of Oregon Brain Development Lab. This DVD is aimed at general audiences.

CHAPTER 2

Making Connections: How Brain Cells and Regions Communicate

"The brain is like a muscle. When it is used, we
feel very good! Understanding is joyous."
Carl Sagan. *Broca's Brain.* 1979.

CHAPTER ONE SHOWED THAT EXPERIENCE INFLUENCES BRAIN
cells to connect, changing the brain's structure. This chapter
describes how brain cells—specifically, tiny neurons invisible to
the naked eye—make these connections. In addition, it discusses
how larger regions, especially the cortex, enable us to function and
make us human.

An understanding of how neurons connect and of how regions
behave reminds us that the human brain is a work in progress, at
once vulnerable and full of potential. Once we know how neurons
join together and how regions interact, we feel compelled to ask
conscientiously and often, "What shall I do today to weave circuits
in my own brain? What shall I do to affect the development of
circuitry in children's brains? What behavior will help the elderly
strengthen their brains?"

Two kinds of brain cells

As we noted briefly in chapter one, the brain consists of two kinds of brain cells: neurons (nerve cells) and glial cells. Neurons are the brain's powerhouse. They generate words, thoughts, feelings, and actions. Without the help of glial cells, however, this powerhouse would not operate smoothly and efficiently. In fact, new research suggests that glial cells perform roles only now beginning to be understood and deserve credit for most of the brain's work.[1]

It has long been known that over ninety percent of all brain cells are glial cells. The word "glial" comes from the Greek "glia" for "glue." These cells are aptly named because their primary job is to support and assist—to be the metaphorical "glue"—for neurons. On the one hand, we are born with a specific allotment of neurons. On the other hand, glial cells divide and increase as they are needed. The more connections neurons make, the more glial cells the brain produces.

Just as a hospital's staff performs a variety of jobs, so glial cells—there are six varieties—serve and aid neurons by performing many tasks.[2] For instance, glial cells fit into spaces around neurons to hold neurons together in a multitude of complex structures. Far from being randomly scattered throughout the brain, neurons are arranged in intricate columns, rows, layers, and clusters. Glial cells hold these arrangements in place. Glial cells also feed and nourish neurons. Astrocytes, for example, are star-shaped glial cells that, among other things, cause blood vessels in the brain to expand or contract. By connecting to these blood vessels and influencing whether they shrink or enlarge, the astrocyte glial cell manages the delivery of oxygen and nutrients to neurons. In addition to feeding neurons, glial cells eat invading viruses and bacteria, mop up and remove potentially toxic chemicals that gather around neurons, get rid of dead neurons, and form scars to wall off brain tumors.

A variety of glial cell known as the oligodendrocyte functions to myelinate axons in the central nervous system. That is, it wraps myelin, a white fatty substance, around the neuron's axon, a single thin fiber that carries the neuron's out-going signal. Myelin is comparable to plastic insulation wrapped around an electric wire to increase its efficiency. It insulates the axon fiber so that it can transmit its signal rapidly and easily. Multiple sclerosis, an autoimmune disease, attacks both the neuron's myelin and the glial cells that produce myelin. When myelin disappears, the axon that it protects dies, along with the neuron itself.

Glial cells aid and support neurons not only from birth to death, but even before birth.[3] To construct the developing brain *in utero,* neurons migrate to the places in the brain they are meant to occupy. Their migration is possible because glial cells precede them. Setting off ahead of the neurons, glial cells assume the form of a rope or vine. Neurons follow, sliding along this glial rope until they arrive at the point in the developing brain that they are meant to occupy. Reaching this point, the neurons drop off. If glial cells did not provide a pathway for neurons to follow, the neurons could not migrate.[4] Glial cells make certain that neurons survive and function normally.

The elegant neuron

Although the importance of glial cells cannot be exaggerated, neurons are the stars of the nervous system. Over one hundred and fifty different kinds of neurons enable us to breathe, feel, think, aspire, and love, for they alone among the body's cells are capable of firing electrical signals. The neurons in an average brain generate about twelve watts of electricity, enough to power a small flashlight. Neurons transmit not only electrical, but also chemical signals. It is these electro-chemical signals that make possible all brain functioning. Exactly how the signaling occurs deserves close attention. We begin by identifying the neuron's parts.

The neuron's three parts

A neuron consists of three parts: the cell body, dendrites, and one axon. All these parts are contained within the cell's membrane, the tissue that makes the cell a separate unit. The cell body, or *soma* (Greek for "body"), contains everything the neuron needs to live, such as a nucleus that holds DNA, energy-producing mitochondria, special structures involved in making proteins, and ions— atoms that have gained or lost an electron. A tiny fraction of the size of the period at the end of this sentence, the cell body may have one of various possible shapes, such as triangular, oval, round, candelabra, or spindle-shaped.[5]

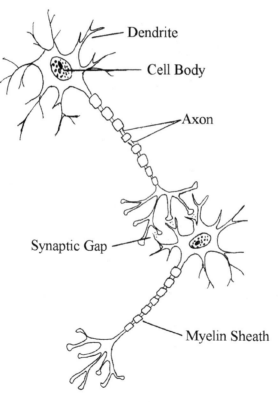

FIGURE 2

The receptive dendrite

Unlike other cells in the human body, neurons possess two kinds of fibers: dendrites and axons. Dendrites (Greek for *tree*) are short, stubby, branch-like fibers about a millimeter long that grow out of the cell body. The primary job of dendrites is to receive signals from other neurons. Dendritic spines, minute protuberances that grow out of the dendrite to enlarge its surface, share in this work. One neuron can possess as many as ten thousand dendrites that receive signals simultaneously from as many as ten thousand to one hundred thousand separate neurons.

Should a dendrite receive a strong excitatory chemical message from another neuron (neurons send messages that either excite or inhibit), that chemical message triggers the dendrite to send its own electrical charge. The electrical charge passes to the cell body and, if the signal is strong enough, through the cell body to the axon, causing the axon to transmit a signal that connects with the next neuron.

When neurons connect, their dendrites grow like trees in sunshine, becoming bushier and more elaborate. Dendrite branches grow longer, spread out, split in two, and grow more spines.

When this happens, the surface of the neuron from which these fibers extend increases. As the neuron's surface increases, more space is available for that neuron to connect with other neurons. In other words, when neurons connect, causing dendrites to grow, the dendritic growth enlarges neurons and strengthens the brain. No connection would occur, however, were it not for the axon.

The singular axon

Although a neuron has thousands of short, stubby dendrites whose job is to receive signals, it has only one axon. The axon carries outgoing electrical-chemical charges to other neurons. It "acts on" these neurons. As Dr. Susan Greenfield says, "Appearing highly purposeful, yet with the fragility of spun sugar, moving . . . with alarming speed while almost literally feeling their way by means of fluted, web-like endings that undulate and flutter as they make their inexorable progress,"[6] axons seek their target neurons. The electrical charge an axon carries, called the *action potential,* in combination with chemical processes that occur at the end of the axon, make it possible for one neuron to communicate with another.[7]

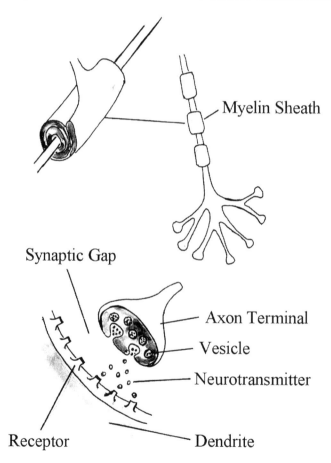

Myelin Sheath

Synaptic Gap

Axon Terminal

Vesicle

Neurotransmitter

Receptor

Dendrite

FIGURE 3

Depending on their location, axons vary in length from 1/1000th of an inch—just long enough to reach neurons in a small cluster—to almost three feet, long enough to extend from a motor neuron down the spinal cord to the foot.[8] At its tip, the axon splits into many terminals, like fingers at the end of an arm. Some axons end in a few terminals, and others in several thousand.

The entire axon carries its electrical charge efficiently because of its myelin sheath. Myelin, a white substance that coats the approximately three million miles of axons in the average human brain, is laid down in cylinders separated by small gaps. Because myelin surrounds axons in the infant's brain stem, an infant's heartbeat, body temperature, and reflexes function efficiently from the moment of birth. Myelin coating also facilitates the infant's control of face, limbs, and trunk.

As the baby develops, more axons acquire myelin, thanks to the work of the oligodendrocyte glial cell. About two months before the child begins to speak, for instance, the part of the brain connected with speech receives myelin. At the age of two, a child's cerebellum, a brain region that influences coordination and balance, becomes myelinated. The cerebellum's myelination gives two-year olds increased coordination. The myelination process takes time. Between the ages of fifteen and the late twenties, for example, myelin slowly covers axons in the prefrontal cortex, the seat of thinking, remembering, paying attention, getting organized, and controlling emotions. One of the main causes of the increased weight of the human brain after birth is the coating of more and more axons with myelin. Once an axon receives its white myelin coating, it looks as white as porcelain and is known as "white matter."[9]

The electrical part of the neuron's electrical-chemical signal

The axon's electrical charge, or action potential, is the product of activity that begins in the cell body. Thousands of dendrites protrude from the neuron's cell body, searching for chemical messages delivered by other neurons. Neurons send two basic kinds of messages, those that excite and those that inhibit. If dendrites receive a message that excites, they pass it on to the neuron. The receiving neuron then generates an electrical charge. If a message inhibits, however, the receiving neuron reduces the charge, producing a state of rest.

A neuron is in a state of rest when it is just sitting there, not firing. In that state of rest, the area inside the cell's membrane is balanced against the area outside. Potassium, sodium, and other ions—charged atoms that have lost or gained an electron—sit inside and outside the cell's membrane, occupying both intercellular and extracellular areas. Tiny channels provide passageways, however, from inside the cell body through the cell's membrane to the outside. These channels make it possible for ions to travel in and out of a neuron. As long as these channels receive sparse and carefully controlled traffic, the neuron remains at rest.

If a sending neuron fires a powerful signal, this signal enters and stimulates the dendrite of the receiving neuron. This stimulation causes ion channels to open in the receiving cell's membrane. These open channels allow positive sodium ions to rush inside the cell, carrying their positive charge. More and more sodium moves in, until finally the inside of the cell becomes more positively charged than the outside. Rest is upset. In this state of inequilibrium, the receiving neuron produces its peak voltage. After the charge hits its peak voltage, potassium ions begin to leave the inside of the membrane. When they move rapidly through the channel to the outside of the membrane, a state of rest is restored.

In other words, one neuron can excite another enough to cause the receiving neuron's ions to change places. When a neuron's ions change places by traveling through membrane channels, a positive-negative wave of electricity, an electrical charge,[10] is produced. This electrical charge eventually affects the axon's terminals in ways that prompt neurons to connect at the synaptic gap.

The synapse

The transmission process that connects two neurons is both electrical and chemical. The process begins with an electrical charge, as we have seen, and ends when two neurons join at a point called the synapse.

Synapse derives from the Greek word "to join together." The term refers to the physical junction—the gap, or cleft—between the axons of one neuron and the dendrites of another. It also refers to the joining together of two neurons. A synapse takes place when two neurons connect at the synaptic gap.

Neurons do not connect by touching and becoming welded together. Were they welded together, they would be rigid, inflexible and incapable of rewiring. The brain's plasticity is indebted to the perpetual separation of neurons. Neurons are always separated by a gap about a millionth of an inch wide. This gap, the "synaptic gap," separates the axon terminals of one neuron from the dendrites of another, as a river separates one side of town from the other.

When a neuron produces an electrical charge and sends it hurtling down its single axon at 220 miles per hour, it intends that the axon should carry that electrical signal to a particular target neuron. When the electrical charge reaches the axon's terminals, however, it can go no further. The synaptic gap, filled with salty, watery fluid, prevents the electrical charge from reaching its destination. To appreciate this interruption, imagine that you are speeding in your red convertible down a country road with the intention of visiting a friend who lives on the other side of the river. You discover that the old covered bridge has collapsed and that only a boat can get you to the other side. Always resourceful, you find a boat, cross the river, and reach your friend's house.

In the same way, the electrical charge is stopped by the salty, watery synaptic gap and must find an alternative way to proceed. Unable to enter the liquid that fills the synaptic gap, the determined electrical charge turns its force on the packets, called vesicles, that are stored in the axon's terminals. These packets contain chemical molecules. The electrical signal jolts these packets, causing them first to merge with the axon membrane and then to open. Opening, they spill their contents, chemical molecules called *neurotransmitters*, into the liquid synaptic gap.

An axon can release more than one neurotransmitter. The neurotransmitter's power depends both on its kind—about twenty-five kinds have been identified and many other candidates have been proposed—and on its location in the brain. Just as any letter of the alphabet plays a part in countless words, so one neurotransmitter can have multiple uses, depending on its different locations.

Released from packets and diffused into the liquid-filled synaptic gap, the neurotransmitters rapidly search out dendrites on the target neuron. Their task is to deliver their chemical message to receptors sitting on the spines—protuberances—of these dendrites. Receptors are custom-designed to receive these chemical molecules. A receptor is like a lock waiting for the only key that can open it. Operating like scanners, receptors sit on dendritic spines and search for the specific chemical signal they were made to receive. When the right neurotransmitter enters the dendrite's receptor, like a hand slipping into a glove, a synapse is formed. A circuit is wired. The receptor will then transmit the signal deep into the receiving neuron's cell body.[11]

Some neurotransmitters excite their receiving neurons into action, while others inhibit the receiving neurons. If a neuron is hit repeatedly by one excitatory neurotransmitter, the neuron will fire. If a neuron is hit simultaneously by neurotransmitters from many other brain cells, it will also fire. The excited cell body will open its channels, ions will change places, and a new electrical charge will be generated. Thus the receiving neuron becomes transformed into a sending neuron.[12]

The receiving neuron, called *postsynaptic*, uses only as much of the neurotransmitter as it needs. Its receptors release back into the synaptic gap any unused neurotransmitter. Awash in the gap, the ejected neurotransmitter cannot be allowed to linger. It is either recycled or tossed out as waste. Recycling, called *re-uptake*, occurs when a transporter molecule helps the cast off neurotransmitter return to the axon of the sending (*presynaptic*) neuron. The neurotransmitter re-enters the axon that released it in the first place, and the economical presynaptic axon then repackages the neurotransmitter, placing it in vesicles for future release.

A neurotransmitter that has been ejected by the postsynaptic receptor and that is not helped by a transporter molecule to return to its original axon is removed as waste from the synaptic gap. Enzymes rip the neurotransmitter into little pieces. The pieces then move from the cerebrospinal fluid into the blood stream and from the bloodstream to the bladder, which expels them.[13]

The process described above may be summarized as follows:

1. An electrical charge—an action potential—shoots down the length of the axon to its terminal and jolts open packets holding chemical molecules called neurotransmitters.

2. The neurotransmitters push through the liquid in the synaptic gap to deliver their signals to receptors on the dendritic spines of the target neuron. Most neurotransmitters connect

with receptors on the spines of dendrites, although fifteen to twenty percent of the connections they make are with receptors on the outside of the cell body itself.

3. When the neurotransmitters enter the receptors on the dendrites of the receiving neuron, the neurons connect.

4. If the signal it receives is strong, the receiving (postsynaptic) neuron generates its own electrical charge and sends it on to its neighbor neuron.

Regions

The complex process that enables infinitesimal neurons to join at the synaptic gap inspires awe. Equally remarkable is the way that large regions interact. Each of the brain's regions, composed of billions of neurons and visible to the naked eye, is carefully designed to carry out distinctive functions. No region is able to function, however, without interacting constantly with other regions. The brain is a collaborative enterprise, a system of intricately connected subsystems.

Hemispheres

The brain has two sides, as does the body. These sides, called hemispheres,[14] come together like the two sides of a yo-yo. They sit on top the brain stem, perched on its stalk. The brain stem extends down from the hemispheres through a hole in the skull and attaches to the spinal cord. Without our being consciously aware of it, the brain stem supervises a host of internal processes that keep us alive. It controls such functions as blood circulation, body temperature, heart rate, breathing, and oxygen levels.

The hemispheres, each of which is covered by the cortex, a thin, wrinkled outer layer, are separated by a deep groove called the longitudinal fissure that extends from the nose to the back of the brain.[15] The corpus callosum, a large cable made of about 250,000 axons, connects these two hemispheres, making it possible for them to communicate and share information. Because the two hemispheres do communicate constantly, they act as one, always in concert.[16]

Each hemisphere has its own distinctive functions. The functions of one hemisphere complement and complete those of the other.[17] The *left hemisphere*, for example, is hardwired to use logic, problem solve, understand language and speak. It sees the particular thing, the tree, not the forest, and it is concerned with the meanings of words, not their emotional impact. However, *the right hemisphere* deals not with specific words, but with their rhythm and tone. Indeed, the right hemisphere helps us communicate with others by interpreting tone of voice, reading facial expressions, and recognizing faces. It deals not with musical notes, but with melody. It engages in flights of imagination. Disposed to perceive the whole picture, it sees the ocean, not the particular wave.

Each hemisphere controls the opposite side of the body. The cortex of the right hemisphere controls the movement, for instance, of the left arm and leg, and it handles sensory input from the left ear and hand. The cortex of the left hemisphere controls sensory impulses received from the right hand and the right toes, and movement of the right arm and leg. Because they are in constant communication, the right hemisphere knows what the left is doing. The two cortical hemispheres handle distinctive processes, but because the corpus callosum lets them talk, they act together as a single cohesive unit. Thanks to the corpus callosum, then, we humans do not have a left brain and a right brain; we have one brain.

The cortex

Among the brain's many regions, the cortex, more than any other, makes us human. It is the seat of our intellectual being. It enables us to think, feel, hear, sing a song, plan a trip, and recognize a friend. Because of the cortex, we learn and remember. "Cortex" comes from the Latin word meaning "bark." Just as bark covers a tree, so the cortex covers the hemispheres. It encases the brain's mass, varying in thickness from 1/32 to ¼ of an inch. It is also deeply wrinkled, like a walnut, from being pressed together to fit inside the skull's limited space. The ridges in the wrinkled surface are called "gyri" (singular "gyrus") and the grooves are called "sulci" (singular "sulcus"). "Fissure" is the term given to very deep grooves. If the cortex were spread out and ironed flat, it would cover about two and a half square feet, about the size of a newspaper page. The cortex is called "gray matter," but it only looks gray in a dead brain.[18] In living brains, it looks "like those rivers that run reddish-grayish-brown after a thunderstorm."[19]

The entire cerebral cortex consists of six layers. Six sheets of neurons are stacked on top of one other. The individual neurons in one sheet are designed to line up with the neurons in the sheets directly above and below. In this way, the neurons form columns. These vertical columns, which cut through all six sheets and are the thickness of a spider's web, seem to organize themselves around similar interests, "like a club that self-organizes out of a crowd at a party, where people of similar interests tend to cluster together."[20] These vertical columns connect with one another, thus generating great complexity.[21]

The six cortical layers do more than provide vertical columns. Each layer is unique. Neurons in the deepest layers, for instance, serve mainly as an outbox, carrying messages out of the cortex to distant subcortical structures such as the thalamus or spinal cord.

Neurons in the middle layers of the cortex are like an inbox; they receive messages from the thalamus and other areas. The layers closest to the surface are like an "interoffice box; they make . . . connections with the superficial layers of other regions...."[22]

In the cortex, cell bodies converge to form what is called "gray matter." Extending from these cell bodies are axons. Some of these axons operate only in one hemisphere, connecting with neurons in various areas of that single hemisphere. Other axons cross from one hemisphere to the other, connecting neurons in both hemispheres. Still other axons run up and down to connect various groups of neurons.

The Four lobes: frontal, temporal, parietal, occipital

Each hemisphere of the cortex is divided anatomically into four physical lobes, or sections—the frontal, temporal, parietal and occipital lobes. Although both hemispheres contain these four lobes, it is customary to refer to the lobes in the singular, as if only one of each kind existed.[23]

The frontal lobe

The frontal lobe, occupying one third of the entire cortex, takes up more real estate than do other lobes. Containing the prefrontal cortex, the premotor cortex, and the motor cortex, the frontal lobe accounts for many of the qualities peculiar to human beings. This lobe extends from behind the nose to the central fissure, a deep groove running from ear to ear.

The central fissure separates the frontal lobe from the parietal lobe, which is located directly behind it. If we trace the frontal lobe from the central fissure towards the forehead, we first encounter the motor cortex, the area of the cortex that begins a movement. It is the area that starts the quarterback's passing action. Parallel

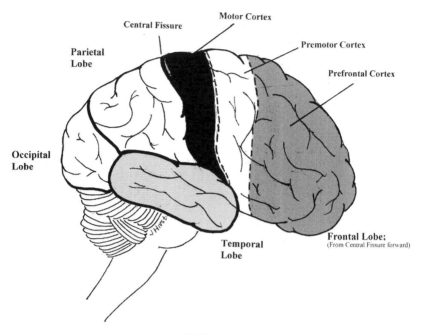

FIGURE 4

to, and in front of, the motor cortex is an area called the premotor cortex. The premotor cortex is busy before the motor cortex engages. Its work precedes that of the motor cortex. It plans the quarterback's pass. Only afterwards does the motor cortex launch the football. With the cerebellum's help, the football reaches the targeted receiver.

Extending from the premotor cortex to the forehead is the prefrontal cortex, the part of the brain that makes us unique. The prefrontal cortex, located just behind the forehead, is "the only part of the brain that is free from the constant labour of sensory processing."[24] It does not concentrate on interpreting nerve impulses that reach it from the senses. Instead, the prefrontal cortex has the spectacular job of wiring circuits that hold our developing personality, control emotions, and curtail impulsive actions. Referred to as the brain's CEO, the prefrontal cortex anticipates the future, formulates objectives, plans, organizes, and evaluates. It judges, decides, imagines, and solves problems. In addition, it is the seat of our working memory, and it wires circuits for social intelligence.[25]

The frontal lobe not only performs all the functions of the prefrontal lobe, premotor cortex, and motor cortex. In addition it is hardwired for other operations, including speech. A place in the left frontal lobe, by the left temple, lets people articulate words. Thanks to this area, discovered in 1861 by Frenchman Paul Broca and known as Broca's area, we are able to string words together and pronounce sentences.

The temporal lobe

In 1871 Austrian Carl Wernicke discovered an area in the left temporal lobe that also contributes to human speech. Labeled "Wernicke's area," this area is hardwired to let us understand language, think about it, and formulate coherent statements. This part of the temporal lobe lets people understand the meanings of the words they hear. Those who suffer damage to Wernicke's area hear words as clicks and grunts and formulate sentences that sound like gibberish.[26]

The findings of Wernicke and Broca show that our use of language depends upon the interaction of the brain's various regions. Because Wernicke's area in the temporal lobe cooperates with Broca's area in the frontal lobe, as well as with various other areas in the cortex that handle other aspects of language like verbs and prepositions, human beings possess language. The brain is a system of numerous regions, or subsystems, that need each other.

In addition to Wernicke's area, the temporal lobe, situated just behind the temples and above the ears, also contains the auditory cortex, the cortical area that receives and interprets information about sound. The auditory cortex lets us hear the wind blowing and figure out what it means. It decides if the wind sounds like a gentle breeze or a hurricane. If the tree fell in the woods and no auditory cortex were present to receive and interpret sound waves and assign meaning to nerve impulses, the tree would make no sound.

The versatile left temporal lobe also participates in the *What* system. Stored in the temporal lobe, in

> "Stored in the temporal lobe ... is information that identifies what an object is....The parietal lobe identifies where in space an object is located....The Where and What systems cooperate to assure our safe passage."

its neural networks, is information that identifies what an object is. Until information reaches the temporal lobe to be interpreted, the brain does not know what it is looking at. Consider what happens when you look at a pink carnation. Sensory information travels from your retina to the visual cortex in the occipital lobe at the back of the brain. This visual cortex breaks down the pink carnation and maps its features—color, shadow, diagonal line—onto various neurons. Some neurons react to its pink hue, others to the flower's shape, and others to yet different features. Although the visual cortex dissects and analyzes the pink carnation, it does not know what it is. To know what the carnation is, the brain must compare it with the shapes of other objects it has seen. Memories of the shapes the brain has seen are stored in the temporal lobe. A neural pathway carries information about the pink carnation from the visual cortex in the occipital lobe to the temporal lobe. When the temporal lobe receives the features of the pink carnation, it compares them with shapes it knows. This comparison enables your brain to tell you that you are seeing a pink carnation.

The next question is, "Where is that carnation located?" To

answer this question, the brain's *What* system needs help from its *Where* system, which is located in the parietal lobe.

The parietal lobe

The parietal lobe sits at the top of the head and immediately behind the central fissure—the deep groove crossing from ear to ear—that separates the parietal lobe from the frontal lobe. Like other areas of the cortex, it aids thinking. It also processes touch, pain, pressure, and spatial awareness. At the very front of the parietal lobe is an area designated the "somatosensory" cortex. This area processes sensory information about the body—such as pain from a cut on the arm, or pressure from a handshake, or the feel of soft velvet.

The parietal lobe also contains the *Where* system. The parietal lobe identifies *where* in space an object is located. The *Where* system tells us if an object is close, far away, behind, to the right or to the left. It also identifies an object's motion. If the object is moving, the parietal cortex tells us how fast it is going and in what direction. Damage to part of the parietal lobe makes it impossible to judge an object's location or its motion. Those with such damage cannot tell how close they are to a cliff's edge or how near they are to the top step of a steep staircase. To be safe, they are obliged to avoid cliffs and stairs.[27] They must also give up walking across the street because to them moving cars seem frozen in space.

The *Where* and *What* systems cooperate to assure our safe passage. The parietal lobe's *Where* system, for instance, reveals where the tree is located in relation to the skier's body—straight ahead on the slope—so that the skier can avoid colliding with it. The *What* system in the temporal lobe tells the skier what he has seen—a tree. The frontal lobe contemplates the meaning of what he sees. Working together, these distinct regions get the skier safely down the mountain.

The occipital lobe

Like the parietal and temporal lobes, the occipital lobe also performs various distinctive functions. Located at the very back of the head, behind the temporal and parietal lobes, it contains the visual cortex. The process of vision begins when the eye carries light waves to the retina. The retina absorbs light rays and transmits this information as sensory nerve impulses from the retina along the optic nerve to a subcortical structure called the thalamus. From the thalamus, signals travel to the visual cortex in the occipital lobe. As we noted above, different neurons in the visual cortex are hardwired to react to particular nerve impulses. One set of neurons is wired to respond to the color red, for instance, and another to diagonal lines. The visual cortex sends these signals to the temporal lobe, so that the brain can figure out what an object is, and to the parietal lobe, so the brain can tell where an object is located, and to the frontal lobe, so the brain can discern the object's meaning.[28]

When the visual cortex in the occipital lobe registers that you have seen a helicopter, for instance, it needs the temporal lobe to tell you what it is, and the parietal lobe to tell you where the helicopter landed. The frontal lobe thinks about the significance of the helicopter's landing in that place.

This brief view of the brain's cortex indicates the uniqueness and yet interdependence of the brain's different lobes. Like members of a baseball team who play different positions with great independence and at the same time collaborate, so parts of the cortex fulfill distinctive roles, yet collaborate to allow the brain to function.[29] The same cooperation characterizes subcortical structures—those parts of the brain below the cortex.

Subcortical structures

If a hemisphere were transparent so that we could look through its side to its interior, we would see several structures below the cortex. Each hemisphere contains the same structures, although neuroscientists refer to these structures in the singular. In each hemisphere, for example, organized around the top of the brain stem, are the thalamus and hypothalamus. The thalamus, which means *inner chamber* or *ante-room,* is the area to which nerve impulses from the senses must report. The thalamus then dispatches these sensory impulses to appropriate parts of the cortex for analysis. The hypothalamus, located below the thalamus, keeps the body balanced. If your temperature soars, for example, the pearl-size hypothalamus tries to bring it down. The hypothalamus reminds you to eat and tells you when you are thirsty. Among many other functions, it also initiates a neural pathway that culminates in the production of stress hormones that affect heart rate, breathing, and blood pressure.

The cerebellum

Located at the base of the brain is a fist-shaped structure known as the cerebellum, or "little brain." This region is responsible for the coordination of external movements and learned motor skills. When you turn in your chair, reach for a coffee cup on the table and bring it back to your lips, all the while sitting erect, your cerebellum is responsible. It governs your movements and maintains your balance. After you mastered the art of riding a bicycle, the cerebellum let you ride without thinking about it. The cerebellum makes it possible for an artist to draw an exact image of the young man riding his skateboard and for a preschooler to color inside the lines.

To coordinate movement, the cerebellum collaborates with the motor cortex. It is able to communicate with the motor cortex because a small structure known as the pons, a name meaning "bridge," acts as a bridge linking the cerebellum to the cortex. Recent experiments suggest that the cerebellum may also cooperate with other brain regions to do more than coordinate physical movement. It may also help us order our thoughts into sequences. We think up a plan—a way to make the luggage fit into the car—and then act to carry it out. Perhaps the cerebellum helps us order the steps in that plan. Neuroscientists are finding evidence to suggest that the same brain circuits that order steps in a physical activity may also help order and sequence a mental act.[30]

Conclusion

Although myriad subcortical structures exist, many of which are discussed in later chapters, these few examples help convey the idea of a highly integrated brain. Subcortical regions and cortical lobes interact in countless ways, just as neurons constantly work together. The result of the interrelatedness of the brain's regions and neurons is a magnificently complex system of subsystems that allows us to live, breath, move, learn, remember, think, feel, and create the future.

Chapter 2: Endnotes

1. For new information about the operation of glial cells, see R. Douglas Fields, "The Hidden Brain," *Scientific American Mind* (May/June 2011), pp. 53-59.

2. Rita Carter, *Mapping the Mind* (Berkeley: University of California Press, 1998), p. 14; Michael S. Sweeney, *Brain: The Complete Mind* (Washington D. C.: National Geographic, 2009), p. 10; Katherine Leitzel, "The Other Brain Cells," *Scientific American Mind* (June/July, 2008), p. 7. Among kinds of glial cells are oligodendrocytes, which form myelin; microglia, which detect damaged or unhealthy neurons and eat foreign invaders such as bacteria and viruses; and astrocytes, which hold neurons in place, feed them and clean up dead neurons. It may be that neurons are somehow involved in processing information, but research has not confirmed this. For discussion of how neurons connect, see Greenfield, pp. 45-100.

3. Susan A. Greenfield, *The Human Brain: A Guided Tour* (New York: Basic Books, 1997), pp. 4, 99; Robert Sylwester, *A Celebration of Neurons: An Educator's Guide to the Human Brain* (Alexandria, VA: Association for Supervision and Curriculum Development, 1995), pp. 29-30.

4. Marian Diamond and Janet Hopson, *Magic Trees of the Mind* (New York: Plume Book, 1999), pp. 44-47; 15-20.

5. David A. Sousa, *How the Brain Learns* (Reston, Virginia: NASSP, 1995), p. 4. William H. Calvin, *How Brains Think: Evolving Intelligence Then and Now* (New York: Basic Books, 1996), p. 115; Greenfield, 66-70.

6. Greenfield, p. 111.

7. Sousa, pp. 1-23; Diamond and Hopson, pp. 26-27.

8. Greenfield, pp. 66-78; Sylwester, pp. 29-30; Sweeney, pp. 11-12; Steven Hyman, "Susceptibility and 'Second Hits,'" in *States of Mind*, ed. Roberta Conlan (New York: The Dana Press and John Wiley & Sons, 1999), pp. 9-16; Richard Restak, *The Secret Life of the Brain* (New York: The Dana Press and the Joseph Henry Press, 2001), pp. 8-9. Sylwester, p. 33.

9. Calvin, p. 115.

10. Robert M. Sapolsky, *Biology and Human Behavior: The Neurological Origins of Individuality, 2nd edition,* (Chantilly, Virginia: The Teaching Company, 2005), pp. 9-18; Greenfield, pp. 66-72; Sapolsky lecture given in Portland, Oregon, for the OHSU Brain Awareness Lecture Series, February 5, 2003; On the movement of positively charged sodium and potassium ions through a neuron's cell membrane, see Rita Carter, Susan Aldridge, Martyn Page, Steve Parker, *The Human Brain Book* (London: DK Publishers, 2009), p. 72.

11. Calvin, pp. 115-118; Steven Hyman, "Susceptibility and 'Second Hits,'" in *States of Mind*, ed. Roberta Conlan (New York: John Wiley & Sons, Inc.) 1999, pp. 12-15; Diamond and Hopson, pp. 21-26; One neuron reacts to input from thousands of cells. Greenfield, pp. 78, 80, 83: When the target cell sends its signal to a neuron, its signal will "become one of thousands impinging on yet the next target cell." As many as from ten thousand to one hundred thousand neurons simultaneously make contact with any particular target neuron. They send "different chemicals" to the receptors of dendrites; see also Sylwester, pp. 29-30.

12. Joseph LeDoux, *The Emotional Brain* (New York: Simon & Schuster, 1996), p. 214; Sweeney, pp. 14-16; Sapolsky, *Biology and Human Behavior* pp. 9-37; Greenfield, pp. 66-81; Sylwester, pp. 33-39; David Sousa, pp. 4, 5, 32.

13. Sapolsky, *Biology and Human Behavior,* pp. 9-37; Greenfield, pp. 66-81.

14. Although some neuroscientists equate the two hemispheres with the brain's two sides, others equate it with the two halves only of the cortex. Strictly speaking it is the right side

of the cortex that controls the left side of the body, and vice versa. NINDS, the National Institute of Neurological Disorders and Strokes, defines "hemisphere" as "cerebrum." See Ninds.nih.gov/disorders/brain_basics/know_your_brain.htm

15. *Fissure* is the name given to deep grooves, and *sulcus* (plural *sulci)* is the name given to small grooves. The *gyrus* is a ridge, or bump. Many ridges, *gyri,* occur between fissures.

16. On cortex, hemispheres, lobes, see, Carter, pp. 16, 35-39; 115, 121; John P. J. Pinel with Maggie Edwards, *A Colorful Introduction to the Anatomy of the Human Brain* Boston: Allyn and Bacon, 1998), pp. 68-69; 106-110; Diamond and Hopson, pp. 15-20; Sweeney, pp. 123; 42; Esther Sternberg, *The Balance Within* (New York: W. H. Freeman and Company,2001), pp. 28-38. Norbert Herschkowitz and Elinore Chapman Herschkowitz, *A Good Start in Life* (New York: Dana Press, 2004), pp.128-130; Goldberg, pp. 35-42; Daniel Goleman, *Emotional Intelligence* (New York: Bantam Books, 1995), p. 11; Sylwester, pp. 47-56; Greenfield, p.15; Norman Doidge, *The Brain that Changes Itself* (New York: Viking, 2007), p. 226.

17. Sweeney, pp. 21, 39, 70-71; 123.

18. Greenfield, p. 14. The cortex contains hollows (ventricles) filled with fluid. This cerebrospinal fluid, among other things, nourishes tissues and cushions the brain. When dead cell bodies are pickled in a jar, they have a gray hue.

19. Calvin, p. 115.

20. Calvin, p. 118.

21. Daniel J. Siegel, *The Mindful Brain* (New York: W.W. Norton & Co., 2007), p. 36.

22. Calvin, pp. 117-118.

23. For the distinction between structural lobes and functional cortical areas see Michael Gazzaniga, *Human* (New York: HarperCollins Books, 2008), p. 18-23.

24. Carter, p. 182.

25. Like virtually all CEO's, the prefrontal cortex has an administrative assistant. The administrative assistant is the anterior cingulate cortex, hardwired to decide what incoming information should be passed on to the prefrontal cortex for its attention and deliberation.

26. Thomas Lewis, Fari Amini, Richard Lannon, *A General Theory of Love* (New York: Vintage, 2000), pp. 58-59.

27. On What and Where Systems see Vilayanur S. Ramachandran and Diane Rogers-Ramachandran, "I See, But I Don't Know," *Scientific American Mind* (December 2008/ January 2009), pp. 20-22; Sharon Begley, *Train Your Mind, Change Your Brain* (New York: Ballantine Books, 2007), p. 81; Joel Davis, *Mapping the Mind* (Secaucus, N.J.: Birch Lane Press, 1997), pp. 122-125; LeDoux, *The Emotional Brain* (New York: New York: Simon & Schuster, 1996), pp. 76-78. "Different . . . functions are localized in different regions of the brain....each [brain] area functions by way of the system of which it is a part.. . . Functions are mediated by interconnected systems of brain regions working together rather than by individual areas working in isolation."

28. Greenfield, pp. 40-49.

29. Greenfield, pp. 30-31; See Caviness Jr., et al. *Cerebral Cortex* (August, 1998) pp. 372-384: The percentage of total cerebral cortex volume in humans: frontal lobe=41%; temporal lobe=22%; parietal lobe=19%; occipital lobe=18%.

30. John Ratey, *A User's Guide to the Brain* (New York: Vintage, 2002), pp. 148-149.

CHAPTER 3

Memory and Emotion

"Nothing is so much strengthened by practice,
or weakened by neglect, as memory."
Quintillian. *Institutio Oratoria,* tr. John S. Watson. 1856.

"The energy that actually shapes the
world springs from emotions."
George Orwell, in H. L. Hart, *Why Don't We Learn from History?*

THE EIGHTEENTH-CENTURY WRITER SAMUEL JOHNSON SAID, "Memory is the primary and fundamental power, without which there could be no other intellectual operation."[1] Memory revives the past and gives meaning to the present. It lets us recognize friends and family, recite lines from Shakespeare's *Hamlet,* and find the way home from the grocery store. Memory lets us recall our name, password, social security number, and address. It preserves events and weaves them into an autobiography. Thanks to memory, every human being has a personal story to tell. Understanding how memory works—its location, the link between working memory and long-term memory, and the influence of emotion and meaning on things we remember helps us strengthen our own ability to recall events and information.

Location of memory

Scientists once thought that long-term memories existed in one specific part of the brain. Today they agree that no single structure in the brain is the seat of memory. The brain does not pack the memory of a journey to Antarctica and the memory of the plot of *To Kill a Mockingbird* into a warehouse reserved only for memories. There is no special place in the brain that holds the memory of the first car you ever owned. Instead, the brain scatters features of that first car throughout many regions. In one part of the brain, a set of neurons stores the car's color. In another area, a group of neurons stores the feel of the dashboard. Another group of neurons holds the smell of upholstery. Another circuit holds the sound of the engine, and still other neural circuits in different parts of the brain retain events and emotions that you associate with your first car.

Just as information about a first car is located in neural circuits dispersed in different regions of the brain, so the size, shape, color, softness, and smell of the family's black Labrador retriever, along with emotions and episodes involving the dog, are located in many brain regions. Interestingly, the specific circuit that holds the color black participates in memories of all things black, such as black coal or a black roof. In this it is comparable to the alphabet's letter "s." That single "s" occurs in a multitude of different words. The brain, reflecting nature's propensity to create rich ends from simple means, uses economical bits of information held in a specific group of neurons to recall a profusion of diverse memories.

As these examples of the car and the dog suggest, memories reside in pathways of connected cells.[2] First, an experience stimulates and strengthens connections between neurons,[3] thereby forming a neural pathway and causing us to learn: *neurons fire together*. When the brain keeps this neural circuit—when *neurons wire together*—we remember what we learn.⁴ Once the memory is embedded in a circuit, a neural pathway, then each time one of the neurons in the pattern fires, the others fire. Firing causes a "momentary . . . *replication* of patterns that were once experienced."⁵ Neurons that fire together wire together, becoming a memory.

Why neurons that fire together eventually wire together

The process that wires neurons into a memory is easy to grasp. Suppose that Neuron 1 fires with great power on Neuron 2. Because Neuron 2 receives a repeated and powerful impulse from Neuron 1, Neuron 2 undergoes a chemical change that makes it more excitable. This chemical change is called *long-term potentiation* (LTP). Long-term potentiation causes receptors that normally reside inside the cell body to rise up to Neuron 2's surface, where they stand prepared to receive another signal. Neuron 2 is now excitable, or potentiated. These exposed receptors will stay on the surface in this alert state for hours or days, making Neuron 2 more responsive to stimulation from Neuron 1. If Neuron 1 fires again during this period, even very slowly, or even with a weak signal, Neuron 2 will respond. The more Neuron 1 activates Neuron 2, the more receptive Neuron 2 becomes. Each time the two cells fire together, their synaptic connections are strengthened until eventually Neuron 1 and Neuron 2 are permanently bound together so that when one cell fires, the other fires. Once this bond is established, the slightest signal from Neuron 1 will activate Neuron 2. In other words, the neurons are wired into a circuit. Long-term potentiation has strengthened the synapse between Neuron 1 and Neuron 2. A memory has been formed.⁶

When Neuron 1 and Neuron 2 fire together repeatedly, they develop the energy to activate any neighboring cell to which both are attached. "Cortical neurons are . . . silent unless input conditions are surging—and then their output is proportional to how much they're stimulated."[7] In this way, three neurons become bound together in a distinctive firing pattern. Memory resides in the elaborate circuits, or networks, made by connected neurons. The question remains: How do the senses signal these neurons in the first place, sparking the memory process?

The five senses and brain regions

The brain depends for everything it knows and every skill it possesses on movement and the five senses. These are the brain's only sources of information about the outside world. Each of the five senses transmits signals along hardwired pathways to neurons located in a particular brain region. The more senses we use to learn something, the more we activate neurons in different regions of the brain. Thus the neurons in one region link up with those in other regions to fashion a network that holds a memory. Each

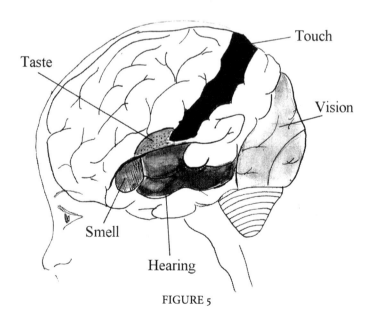

FIGURE 5

group of neurons in this network has the power to re-activate neurons belonging to the same circuit, and re-activation calls up a memory.[8]

Consider how many senses are activated when a young man proposes to his girlfriend. The young couple is savoring prime rib at their favorite restaurant [taste]. The white linen tablecloth shimmers in the reflected light of five scented candles [sight; smell] A violinist serenades the couple with their special song [hearing]. A waiter brings the woman a bouquet of pungent gardenias and carnations, and as she and her date draw near, bending over the bouquet to smell the flowers, their heads gently touch [smell; touch]. Noticing a paper pinned to the bouquet, the woman opens it to find a message from her companion. She reads it aloud, smiles happily, raises her wine glass to him, and slowly sips some wine [hearing, sight, touch, taste]. The man then moves from his chair, gets down on one bended knee, and proposes, offering in his outstretched arm the bright engagement ring. Everyone in the crowded restaurant immediately cheers and applauds.

Years later when this couple celebrates their fiftieth wedding anniversary, the husband and wife will very likely share many memories of this marriage proposal. The reason is that the proposal involved the five senses. Each sense stimulated circuits in distinctive regions of the brain. The slightest jolt to any one of the circuits that was laid down in a particular region will reactivate related circuits in other regions, causing them to fire together again. For example, the smell of a gardenia might act as a "handle" sufficient to re-activate all the synapses, the neural connections, that the couple generated when they dined together long ago. The emotional impact of the proposal also facilitates memory, as a later discussion of emotion shows.

The couple's recall of that distant proposal uses the long-term memory, one of the two kinds of memory that humans possess.

The other kind, once known as short-term memory, neuroscientists now call *working memory*. Working memory and long-term memory systems serve different purposes that help us navigate through life.[9]

Working memory

Located in the prefrontal cortex, which is situated above and behind the eyebrows, working memory "is the ability to *hold information* in the mind over a period of many seconds and to operate on it mentally."[10] It can simultaneously hold five to seven bits of information, but only if these bits pertain to a single task and only briefly. Working memory lasts only a few minutes, because, according to Alan Baddeley, the system it uses differs from systems affecting long-term memory.[11]

The working memory is activated when something in the outside world—when sensory data—gets one's attention. "Attention [is] the ability to *focus* on a particular mental content to the exclusion of others."[12] In the course of a single day, virtually everyone relies countless times on working memory. Imagine that immediately before entering the grocery store with your shopping list in hand, you receive a call on your cell phone asking you to purchase six additional items. Aware that working memory quickly forgets, you rush through the store looking first for those six items. Working memory is the faculty that lets the baker recall for a few minutes the amount of sugar required in the recipe she just read. It lets the weary traveler retain briefly the motel receptionist's elaborate directions to his parking space and room.

The working memory brings together information from many areas of the brain to apply to a single job. Remarkably, it can find and effortlessly recover the information it needs from any site in the brain. The working memory can pull together at the same time, for instance, a sensation, memory, thought, and emotion. Immediate sensations, memories of an event that happened recently or long ago, old beliefs, new ideas, and emotions are all combined simultaneously in the working memory.[13] No dividing line separates them.

To appreciate the working memory's amazing ability to combine different kinds of data, imagine that you are standing on the sidewalk in the dark at six o'clock in the morning shivering with cold and watching the snow settle on your new sports car, resting upside down in the ditch. [*sensations*] You remember the time two years ago when a friend's car hit ice on the same sharp curve and crashed into the same ditch. [*memory*] You decide, "I'll phone my husband and ask him to come. He can take my place, stay with my wrecked car, and wait for the police. I'll drive his car to my office." [*idea, plan*] You feel happy to have figured out that with your husband's help, you will get to work on time. [*emotion*][14] Your happiness was undiminished by the knowledge that, later in the day, the police would arrive at your office to notify you that a driver is never to leave the scene of an accident.

The hippocampus

Unless information first enters the working memory, it can never be transformed into a lasting memory. When the working memory receives information, it activates the hippocampus, the gateway to long-term memory.

The Latin name *hippocampus*, meaning *seahorse*, was assigned to the hippocampus because its shape slightly resembles that of a seahorse. The hippocampus is located in the temporal lobe and connected to the limbic system. It receives signals from the working memory and from other cortical areas. These signals prompt the hippocampus either to keep, or jettison, information it receives. For example, suppose you are studying T. S. Eliot's *The Wasteland* to prepare for a test. If studying this poem bores and confuses you, chances are good that within eighteen to twenty-five hours[15] after learning about *The Wasteland*, your hippocampus will drop seventy to ninety percent of the information you acquired about the subject. If the hippocampus decides to keep the information, it dispatches it to be stored in various parts of the cortex. In fact, the hippocampus returns signals back up to the places in the cortex where they were initially registered. In this way, by talking to the cortex, the hippocampus fixes long-term memories there.[16] The left hippocampus is involved in fixing memories of words and episodes in life. It contributes to a person's on-going autobiography. The right hippocampus, however, is involved in spatial memory. If you get lost easily, blame your right hippocampus.[17]

If the hippocampus did not let us build new memories, we would be trapped in an eternal present. Such was the tragic fate of H.M., a patient whose hippocampus was surgically removed in an attempt to spare him debilitating epileptic seizures. After the surgery, H.M. could not retain any new facts or events. Each time his doctor arrived, H.M. met him as if for the very first time. Because H.M. could not form new memories, he became utterly dependent on others.

TWO KINDS OF LONG-TERM MEMORY: DECLARATIVE AND PROCEDURAL

Declarative long-term memory

Our long-term memories, embedded in circuits that are peppered throughout the brain, are of two kinds, declarative and procedural. Declarative memory is sometimes referred to as *explicit* because its content can be explicitly expressed in words. In words we declare *what* something is or *what happened*. The declarative memory handles two kinds of information, facts and events (episodes). Memories of facts, sometimes called semantic memories, are typically unrelated to personal experience and have no context. Factual (semantic) memories are formed, for instance, when students practice spelling *geography* or recite the name of the man who was British Prime Minister during World War II. Facts are learned intentionally; one sets out to remember them. Stark, isolated facts are hard to retain because they lack personal meaning. It is easier to remember the number of your hotel room than to recall an isolated number because the hotel room means something to you.

Unlike facts, events occur in specific locations at particular times. Their context gives them significance. Because they have personal implications, we remember events (episodes) without consciously striving to do so. Effortlessly, an event enters the long-term declarative memory. The memory of an event includes more than details about the event itself. It also includes the feelings, sensory perceptions, and thoughts that the event triggered when it happened. The more an event sparks powerful feelings or carries strong meaning, the more likely it is that it will become an enduring memory.

Declarative memories—both factual (semantic) and episodic—shift and change over time. They are not permanent records, like a photograph taken at a birthday party or a video recorded for You Tube. When a driver summons up the memory of the head-on collision that happened to him five years ago, his memory becomes vulnerable. Having been recalled, it can now be revised, as if it were being made for the first time. Five years have given the driver new experiences. Without his knowing it, his brain can apply these new experiences to alter features of his initial memory of the accident. Every time someone recalls a memory, it becomes vulnerable—subject to redesign. A memory is "an interpretation, a newly reconstructed version of the original. In addition, as our age and experience change, versions of the same thing evolve....Memory is essentially recon-structive."[18] Recalling last year's elaborate Fourth of July parade means reactivating the circuits in which the parade memory is embedded. Reactivating these circuits gives the brain the opportunity to change them. In this way, declarative memories change over time. Procedural memories, however, do not alter with time.

Procedural Memory

Procedural memory is automatic, unconscious knowledge. For that reason, it is also called *implicit* memory. To acquire a pro-cedural memory—to master an automatic skill or procedure like typing, serving a tennis ball, playing the clarinet, or tap dancing—requires practice. It takes hard work and repetition to reach the point where unconsciously, without putting words to a physical procedure, the body easily executes a skill like figure skating or playing the violin. Stored mainly in the temporal lobe, cerebellum, and the basal ganglia, procedural skills are very robust. Unlike declarative memories, they do not alter when we recall them. Interestingly, procedural memories include many of our auto-matic, nonverbal interactions with people—such as automatically holding open a door or waving to a friend.

Building long-term memories

The urgent question, especially for parents and educators, is "What can we do to help young people build long-term memo-ries?" One important step that helps the brain retain material is to relax. Anyone who has put in long hours reciting and repeat-ing information will be cheered to know that relaxing helps the brain consolidate information into a declarative long-term mem-ory. Consolidation occurs when the brain strengthens neural cir-cuits that experience has already formed until the circuits become durable.[19] Connections between circuits—synapses—grow stronger when a period of focused learning is followed by a complete change of pace. After concentrating for an hour on conjugating Latin verbs, take a break. Turn to an undemanding activity that lets the brain run on idle for a while. Down-time lets the brain work unconsciously to secure an earlier lesson in the long-term memory. Among the factors that lead to eventual consolidation, two of the most powerful are meaning and emotion.

Meaning and long-term memory

When something holds meaning for us, we remember it. The word *meaning* designates *significance* and *purpose*. Human beings search for meaning—for significance and purpose—in everything they do. The will to find meaning motivates them to attend a dinner party, spend the afternoon doing research, or play soccer. The brain has a deep, basic, biological need to find meaning. Disturbed by unexplained

> "When something holds meaning for us, we remember it."

events and randomness, it asks, "Why did that twenty-one year old die in a fatal car accident?" "What difference does my life make?" "Is this job worth doing?" "Does it hold significance?" Because human beings seek meaning in everything, students appropriately ask, "Why do we have to learn this?"

The brain's search for meaning prompts it to look for patterns and order in everything and to create sequences and designs. For example, the brain weaves isolated sounds into recognizable words, and it combines words into sentences that convey meaning. As theoretical neurophysiologist William Calvin says, "Poets combine words in ways that overwhelm us with intense meaning."[20] Looking for meaning, the brain weaves notes into songs, events into stories, and actions into games. It also strings moments together into life, an autobiography that gives us a sense of self.[21]

Creating order and finding patterns helps the brain predict coming events, a feat essential for survival. When something unexpected breaks a familiar pattern, the brain struggles to assign meaning to the unexpected event. It tries to weave it into a new, orderly pattern. For example, if a couple hiking in the densely wooded Cascade Mountains were to come across a stuffed wing-chair blocking their narrow trail, they would speculate about what the chair's presence might mean. Who could have put the chair on the trail, and why? They would want to explain the chair's presence in a way that gives it meaning.[22]

The brain's interpreter seeks meaning

The brain longs so much for meaning that it makes it up. Part of the brain actually serves as an interpreter that strives to find meaning in experience. The interpreter, located in the left temporal lobe, "interprets the inputs we receive every moment and weaves them into stories to form the ongoing narrative of our self-image and our beliefs. . . . It expands on the actual facts we experience to make sense of, or *interpret*, the events of our life."[23] The interpreter assigns meanings to events, ideas, and facts. Undeterred by its own ignorance, the interpreter will explain the inexplicable and impose order on randomness.

Years of research conducted by Michael Gazzaniga and his colleagues on split-brain patients revealed the interpreter's determination to generate order and find patterns. A split brain is one whose two hemispheres have been separated by a surgical procedure that severs the corpus callosum, a bundle of nerves that joins them. Because of the split- brain operation, which is used to control severe epilepsy, the right and left sides of the brain no longer interact with one another.

When the two hemispheres are connected by the corpus

callosum, they are able to work together; they can harmonize their distinctive functions into a unified brain. They keep each other informed of what the other is doing. For example, if the right side of the brain receives from the left eye an image of a red tulip, the right side of the brain sends a message over the corpus callosum that tells the left side, "I see a red tulip." The left side of the brain, which is able to speak, can then name the object.

In a split-brain patient, the severed corpus callosum keeps the hemispheres from exchanging information. They cannot communicate. This means that the right hemisphere, which is not able to initiate speech, is isolated from the brain's speech center, a structure located in the left hemisphere. Cut off from the speech center, the right hemisphere has no way to arrange for its thoughts to be verbalized. However, the inability of the two hemispheres to communicate does not keep the interpreter on the left side of the brain from assigning meaning to events.

Using special equipment, Gazzaniga revealed the sign "walk" only to the split-brain patient's right brain. Because the bridge between the patient's two hemispheres had been severed, the right brain could not tell the left brain that it had read the sign "walk." It did not have a way to convey this information to the left brain. It also lacked the ability to put into words the fact that it had seen the word "walk." Therefore the left side of the brain was unaware that a "walk" sign had been displayed.

When the patient's right hemisphere registered the word "walk," the patient could not say the word "walk," much less explain why he was walking, but he could obey the sign. Therefore he got up and walked. The left side of the brain did not know, of course, that the right side had seen and obeyed a "walk" sign.

While the patient was walking, the doctor asked him why he was walking. The right side of the patient's brain, incapable of formulating speech and reflecting, could not answer this question. The left hemisphere, capable of speech and reflection, did not know the answer to the question. It had not seen the "walk" sign. But instead of saying, "I don't know," the interpreter wanted to give meaning to the walking action. Therefore despite its ignorance of the "walk" sign, the interpreter caused the patient to answer, "I wanted to go get a Coke."[24] The brain invented an answer because it requires meaning. Its left-hemisphere interpreter "seeks patterns, order, and causal relationships."[25] According to Michael Gazzaniga, the brain's left-hemisphere interpreter wants "all incoming information to make sense and mesh with our ongoing idea of ourself."[26]

Meaning changes memories

The brain is so intent on making meaning that unknowingly, without realizing it, "people make up reasons and believe in them."[27] The need for meaning entices the brain not only to make up reasons, but also to revise its memories. Gradually, over time, we edit a memory, change this bit, modify that part, and omit a fragment. Suppose, for example, that seven years ago a friend's wedding was held outdoors on a bright, sunlit summer day. You attended, although you believed the wedding to be a terrible mistake. Now, seven years later, your memory insists that the wedding took place on a rainy, cold, gray, overcast day. Memory has adjusted to suit the meaning that the wedding held for you when it happened.[28]

Memory also fits the person we have become. Our current circumstances influence how we remember a past event. As Joseph LeDoux says, "The state of the brain at the time of recall can influence the way in which the . . . memory is remembered."[29] If today a woman is proud of her achievements, she may want to glorify them by remembering the past as having been harder than it was. Her brain might rearrange memories to make the climb to success look spectacular. She might remember quite sincerely, but incorrectly, that as a fifth-grader, she walked to school through deep snow not two, but four, miles, and that as a university student, she held not one, but three, part-time jobs.

The brain's perpetual quest for meaning suggests why students learn best when they see meaning in the subjects they study. The tedious repetition of disconnected facts that have no bearing on a student's life does not inspire young people to learn and remember. Trivial, pointless busy work does not wire brains to acquire knowledge. According to Harvard professor Daniel Schachter, an authority on memory, "To establish a durable memory, incoming information must be encoded . . . by associating it meaningfully with knowledge that already exists in memory. . . .Suppose that instead of just repeating the . . . number . . . you attempt to make the number meaningful in some way."[30]

Children and adults learn best when they can connect new experiences and information with existing knowledge and skills. We make this connection all the time. When we are given a new task, for instance, how do we react? Immediately we think about things we have done in the past that might prepare us to handle the new assignment. "Let's see. I think I have done something like this before. Last summer I cooked breakfast for fifty. I suppose I can cook breakfast for one hundred and twenty." We derive meaning from connecting new experiences with information already stored in the long-term memory.

Like meaning, emotion is a major route to the long-term memory. Suppose, for instance, that Jack's study group made him happy when they cheered and congratulated him for solving a difficult calculus problem. Jack's happiness will help him remember the complex steps that led to the problem's solution. Joy etches in the track star's brain the experience of being first across the finish line. Buying a shirt becomes memorable when it involves not just calculating cost, but also reacting emotionally to the salesperson's unusual courtesy. Emotion enlarges our experiences.

Emotion

The word *emotion*, from the Latin *movere*, to *move*, involves feelings and the movements that we use to express our inner state. Many of these movements, in the form of gestures, facial expressions, and body language, are universally understood. People everywhere share "four basic emotions—fear, anger, sadness, and joy—and . . . the other emotions are created from combinations of these four . . ."[31] Emotion shades the moment, colors memories as we recall them, influences how we think, affects what we do, and guides our decisions.

The difference between emotion and feeling

Neuroscientists propose various theories to explain precisely what emotion is. According to Joseph LeDoux, an authority on the system that generates fear, "everyone knows what it [emotion] is until they are asked to define it."[32] Increasingly, neuroscientists make a distinction between *emotion* and *feeling*. They use the term *emotion* to refer to the body's state as a result of its having been acted upon by the limbic system. Used in this way, *emotion* is a physiological state precipitated by the limbic system's response to a stimulus. The term *feeling* refers to conscious recognition of this state. To appreciate the difference between emotion and feeling, it helps to know a little about the limbic system.

The limbic system

The limbic system is involved in emotion, learning, and memory. It consists of many structures of various shapes and sizes located in the cortex and in areas beneath the cortex (subcortical areas). These structures are linked to form a kind of circle around the top of the brain stem. For example, the hippocampus, located in the medial part of the temporal lobe, the amygdala—an almond-shaped sub-cortical structure about as big as the distance from your thumb joint to the thumb's tip and located about ¼ inch in from the ears –, and the subcortical hypothalamus are parts of the limbic system. The hypothalamus runs automatic functions and controls the release of hormones; the hippocampus is involved in memory; and the amygdala acts as the brain's emotional center. These areas talk to one another and, in conjunction with other parts of the limbic system, generate a bodily state. The following scenario illustrates how they interact.

Imagine that you are alone in the house. Working in the kitchen at two in the morning, you hear the unmistakable sound of glass shattering upstairs. Instantly your limbic system takes charge of your body. Recognizing danger, the amygdala orders the hypothalamus to prepare you for fight, flight, or freezing in place by sending signals that will cause the release of hormones that make your heart race and your pulse rocket. Meanwhile the amygdala also activates the hippocampus, which assures that you will remember this event. At the same time, the limbic system contacts the frontal cortex, which reasons about and interprets the noise. After the frontal cortex analyzes the experience, and only after, it becomes possible for you consciously to *recognize* your "feeling" and to say, "I am afraid." This conscious recognition is what neuroscientists call "feeling."[33] Feelings, according to Joseph LeDoux, are "a conscious, subjective experience"[34] that we are able to express to others.[35]

Although the distinction between emotion and feeling is gaining ground in neuroscience, for our purposes *emotion* and *feeling* are treated as synonyms that mean "any agitation or disturbance of mind, feeling, passion; any vehement or excited mental state,"[36] the definition of *emotion* in the *Oxford English Dictionary*.

Causes of emotion

Emotions have two primary causes. One cause is external. Virtually anything in the physical environment can generate emotion, such as the sound of a friend's voice, or the sight of a threatening figure lurking in the dark outside a 7-Eleven. Physical sensations like the sight of a cloudless blue sky or the sound of a forlorn melody also carry emotional weight. Another cause of emotion is internal. A thought or memory may give rise to a strong feeling. Remembering a formal dinner in Japan when it was necessary to eat raw sea creatures of various kinds might evoke a feeling of anxiety, while recalling a friend's encouraging words might inspire happiness.

Whatever their cause, emotions are with us all the time, from the instant we wake up in the morning until we fall asleep at night. To be conscious is to experience some kind of emotional tone.

Sometimes the brain stores unconscious, deep-seated emotions that rush unbidden to the surface, taking over our judgment and directing our behavior. For instance, if Mark's new colleague resembles a person who many years ago humiliated him, then Mark may take an instant dislike to his new colleague without realizing that unconscious feelings from the past are shaping his reaction[37] and coloring his judgment.

Linking reason and emotion

Joseph LeDoux, widely respected for his work on the brain's emotional systems, says, "Minds without emotions are not really minds at all. They are souls on ice—cold, lifeless creatures devoid of any desires, fears, sorrows, pains, or pleasures."[38] Human beings could not flourish if, lacking emotion, they had to rely exclusively on cold reason. Fortunately, the brain connects reason to emotion. A two-way path of neurons connects the reasoning frontal lobe, site of rational analysis, with the amygdala, the brain's emotional center.[39] These regions communicate constantly.[40]

The amygdala also registers incoming information from the senses to decide if an experience is safe or dangerous. The experience of a young woman living on a Montana ranch exemplifies the amygdala's role. Frequently, she drives her nineteen year-old, wheel-chair bound brother (given the alias "Jacob" here) out on the range in their Land Rover to shoot rattlesnakes. On one excursion, Jacob shot an enormous rattlesnake and asked his sister, as was his custom, to bring it to him so that he could cut off its rattles. She grabbed what she assumed was a dead snake, only to have it rear back in her hand preparing to lunge forward and strike. Instantly, without thinking, she dropped the snake and ran. Her amygdala had taken over her body to get her out of there fast, well before her reason could assess the situation.[41] The hippocampus at the same time attached memory to that emotional event. It is fortunate that the amygdala takes control of the body's autonomic nervous system when it perceives a threat. Its fast action saves lives.

It is equally fortunate that the amygdala regularly communicates with the frontal cortex. For it is the frontal cortex that reasons about the signals it receives from the amygdala, perceives the need to moderate the emotions that the amygdala generates, and tells the amygdala to calm down. Despite the best efforts of the frontal cortex to temper emotion, emotion often vanquishes reason. It does so because more connections run from the amygdala to the cortex than run in the opposite direction. Thus "the amygdala has a much greater ability to influence the cortex than vice versa."[42]

Emotion's victory may sometimes be beneficial. Say, for instance, that it prompts a judge to feel compassion and empathy and therefore to temper justice with mercy. Emotion's triumph may also be destructive, as when a judge's secret anger defeats reason, producing an unjust legal ruling clothed in reason's garb.

Extreme emotion

Extreme, overpowering emotion is dangerous. Unmodulated by reason, extreme emotion causes us to lose the Self that every person cultivates throughout life. Imagine that a normally pleasant, soft-spoken man is stunned and infuriated when a store manager accuses him of shoplifting. Exonerated almost immediately, nevertheless that evening the normally even-tempered customer rashly phones the store manager at home to rage, shout, and threaten a lawsuit. Stories that illustrate the terrible harm perpetrated by people overcome with emotion permeate the news, of course. A jealous husband stabs his wife. A driver infuriated by a car's slow pace purposely rams the car from behind. Emotion overwhelms not just individuals living private lives, but also politicians and policy makers whom we expect to make decisions based on fact and logic.

Absence of emotion

Just as emotion needs reason's guidance, so reason needs input from the brain's emotional center. Ideally, reason and emotion balance each other. If reason does not receive signals from the amygdala, if it operates without the aid of emotion, the result is disastrous. As Antonio Damasio explains, cold-hearted logic untouched by empathy produces misguided decisions.[43]

An authority on emotion, Damasio describes the condition of a patient he calls Elliot, who lost the ability to feel emotion. Elliot developed a tumor the size of an orange behind his forehead. The surgery successfully removed Elliot's tumor, but it had two dire effects. It significantly damaged Elliot's frontal lobes, and it also severed the connections between the amygdala, the brain's emotional center, and the prefrontal cortex, the area that reasons. Breaking the connection between the prefrontal cortex and the amygdala prevented emotional signals from reaching the prefrontal cortex. As a result, Elliot could no longer recognize his emotions. He lost the ability to experience emotions.

Before surgery, Elliot had been a considerate, affable, responsible family man and employee. After surgery, deprived of the guidance of his emotions, Elliot lost the capacity to socialize appropriately with family, friends, or colleagues. "Without emotions, moral judgments and socialization become difficult if not impossible."[44]

He also lost the ability to make even small decisions, such as what sandwich to eat for lunch or what pen to use. Devoid of emotion, Elliot was no longer Elliot. His personality had changed completely.[45]

Human kind would benefit immeasurably, of course, were emotion and reason to co-exist in perfect harmony. In actuality, reason tries and routinely fails to regulate emotion. As we have seen, emotion regularly swamps reason even in healthy brains primarily because the amygdala sends many more signals to the cortex than the cortex sends to the amygdala. Becoming aware of this physiological condition may inspire us to resist it by intentionally striving to train reason to control emotion.

Emotion and decision-making

The following two versions of the Trolley Problem illustrate the difficulty humans have balancing reason and emotion as they make decisions. The first version heeds reason; the second favors emotion.

Version 1. You are on a bridge watching as an out-of-control train hurtles towards five unsuspecting workers on one track. There is a switch near you that can divert the train onto a different track, where only one worker is standing. Would you divert the train to hit one person in order to save five? This decision is impersonal. You do not know the five workers. All you have to do is throw a switch. Most people answer, "Yes." It's a question of logic. The part of your

"Emotion competes with reason and overcomes it. . . .We are not good at willing our emotions to . . . go away."

brain that reasons, that makes pragmatic decisions—the dorsolateral prefrontal cortex—does the math. It tells you to sacrifice one to save five.

Version 2. You are standing on a bridge watching the train aim at five workers on the track below. There is no way to divert the train. However, standing next to you on the bridge is a massively overweight stranger. If you push the stranger off the bridge and onto the track, he will stop the train. You will kill him, but you will save five workmen. Will you push the stranger off the train? Simple logic says, "Kill one; save five." Reason urges that the end justifies the means. But now the situation is personal. You must yourself do harm to someone standing next to you. Because the issue is personal, it engages the emotions. The medial frontal cortex, the part of the brain that thinks about emotion, is activated, so that it feels bad to push a stranger to his death.[46] Emotion and reason struggle to arrive at a decision. Emotion competes with reason and overcomes it. Most people will not push the stranger. Cold-blooded logic, however, would sanction a purely logical, although heartless, decision.

Another example of how emotion and reason interact to guide behavior is provided by a well-known experiment called the "Ultimatum Bargaining Game" involving sharing. Two players are given a chance to split money. One player is given $100.00 and is invited to propose the split. The other player is allowed to accept or reject the offer. If he rejects it, neither player gets anything. Pure logic says, "Having money is desirable." Therefore one expects the first player to offer the worst possible split. Logic also says, "A little money is better than none." Therefore one expects the second player to take whatever is offered. However, typically players in the experiment defy logic. The person proposing the split, although he knows that keeping as much money as possible makes good sense, frequently offers almost a fifty-fifty sharing, which is illogical.

This equitable split is normally accepted. When the first player offers significantly less than a fifty-fifty split, however, the second player does not think, "A little money is better than none," and accept the offer. Instead he rejects it. The second player's feelings of insult, anger and unfairness trump logical self-interest.[47] Emotions sometimes help us make good decisions, sometimes not.[48] The prefrontal cortex tries to govern emotion with its cultivated values and facts, but has trouble prevailing. We are not good at willing our emotions to diminish or go away.

Emotional intelligence

"To navigate the social [and political] world, we must regulate our impulses and emotions."[49] Feelings must be appropriate to the circumstances. Emotions must be kept in check. We may not be able to control experiencing an emotion, but we must learn to control the intensity and duration of our emotions, subdue moods, resist worry, quiet grief, and find reasons to overcome anger. We must develop, as Daniel Goleman points out in his book *Emotional Intelligence,* the ability to recognize and govern our emotions even in the most trying circumstances.[50]

Governing our emotions presupposes that we are aware of them, think about them as they happen, and keep them under control. If we recognize our feelings, we can control emotion in various ways. One method is to refuse to think about the factors that give rise to an emotion. If an unkind remark hurts your feelings, refuse to think about the remark. Another strategy is to divert attention to something else.

The power of diversion to calm emotion was one of the findings implicit in an experiment conducted by Walter Mischel and his colleagues at the Stanford University nursery. Preschool children were told that they could have one cookie, marshmallow, or toy right away if they wished. They had only to ring a bell, and immediately someone would bring it to them. Or they could have two cookies, marshmallows, or toys, but to get two, they had to wait until a person came back of her own accord to bring the treats. Some children quickly gave in to their longing for a treat and rang the bell. Those who managed to subdue their longing did so by distracting themselves in various ways. They stood in a corner facing the wall, or looked at the ceiling, or closed their eyes, or played a game.

Follow up studies showed that when the children who waited to get two treats became teenagers, they earned higher grades in high school and earned higher SAT scores than did those who, as children, asked for the treat immediately. The implication is that being able to recognize and control one's emotions contributes to success. Perhaps young children should receive training in emotional awareness and management.[51]

The power of our emotions to shape our decisions and the importance of governing our emotions cannot be exaggerated. Teachers have long understood, of course, that when a subject excites young people with hope and enthusiasm, they remember the material. Love also inspires learning and remembering. According to the great Chilean biologist Humberto Maturana, love, which he defines as seeing a "person, being, or thing . . . as a legitimate other in coexistence with oneself," is the "only emotion that expands intelligent behavior."[52]

Fear

Positive emotions help students excel. Negative emotions, on the contrary, interfere with learning and memory. Among negative emotions, fear has been the subject of extensive research. Thanks primarily to the work of Joseph LeDoux, neuroscience can now explain how fear works and why it is such an obstacle to learning. When a person feels threatened, the senses transmit nerve impulses to the thalamus. The thalamus is a relay center. It receives incoming sensory signals from the outside world and then simultaneously relays these signals to the amygdala and the cortex. If a signal involves vision, for example, the thalamus relays information to the part of the cortex that interprets vision. If the sensory signal involves hearing, the thalamus sends information to the auditory cortex. At the same time, the thalamus also transmits this information to the amygdala.

The message from the thalamus reaches the amygdala almost instantly because the pathway from the thalamus to the amygdala is direct, short and fast. On the contrary, the pathway that leads to the amygdala by way of the cortex is long and circuitous. To see how this circuitous pathway works, imagine that you hear a noise. The noise produces nerve impulses that first reach the thalamus. The thalamus then sends the signal to your auditory cortex. The auditory cortex assembles, interprets and analyzes the signal. Only then does it pass the message on to the amygdala, along with an explanation of its meaning. Long before it receives this information from the cortex, the amygdala has already received its fast, immediate signal straight from the thalamus. If the amygdala perceives danger in this signal, it takes charge of the autonomic nervous system and readies the body to freeze, or fight, or take flight.[53] Only later does the cortex deliver its reasoned appraisal of the situation.

Constantly the amygdala examines messages from the thalamus to grasp what the five senses are conveying. As it scrutinizes these messages, it asks, "Is this something to love or something to hate? Something to embrace or something to fear?" Although any emotionally arousing situation can activate the amygdala, Joseph LeDoux has shown that this structure is particularly alert to fear.

The experience of one of my second-year university students

illustrates the amygdala at work. She was studying all night at her desk, her back to the open window, preparing for a final examination. At about 1:30 in the morning, the sound of wind and rain suddenly made her feel uneasy. She went to the window and reached out over the sill to grab the latch so that she could pull the window shut. But as she reached out, her arm brushed across the top of a man's head. Immediately the man jumped up from where he had been crouching in the bushes. The student stood in her bedroom staring at him, frozen, unable to move or speak. When the man saw her reaction, he laughed and then fled into the darkness. The amygdala had caused my student to freeze. Only several seconds after the man ran away did her cortex take charge and tell her to slam and lock the window and close the curtain. Long after it happened, the student remembered this event because fear activated not only her amygdala, but also her hippocampus, thus creating an enduring memory of the episode. Any intense emotion can activate the hippocampus to give us an enduring memory.[54]

What happened to this young woman indicates that when fear activates the amygdala, we cannot think clearly. The activated amygdala tells the body to divert oxygen and glucose from the prefrontal cortex—the thinking part of the brain—to other regions that need oxygen and energy if they are to fight, run, or freeze. Busy increasing heart beat, opening blood vessels, and raising blood pressure, oxygen and glucose do not nourish the frontal cortex so that it can think. Fear makes it virtually impossible to concentrate, pay attention, and reason. Teachers who inspire fear prevent young people from learning.

Stress

Just as fear affects both brain and body, so stress can change our mental and physical state. Any threat to our well-being, however slight, may produce stress. A cause of stress—a stressor—may be physical or psychological. For example, chronic pain, fatigue, hunger, and hypothermia are physical states that cause stress. Psychological stressors include things that diminish self-esteem, such as public humiliation, bullying, and loss of social status. Stress occurs when work compels people to violate their principles, and it occurs when employees must obey arbitrary orders that make no sense. Stress makes people feel out of control and helpless. Worry is a familiar cause of stress.

If stress is short-lived and minor, like worry about being late for dinner or misplacing the car keys, it does no harm. A little stress may even be a good thing; it may help us focus attention on a task and stay alert. Too much stress, however, increases one's susceptibility to disease and, if one is already ill, increases the likelihood that the illness will worsen.[55] If stress endures in the form, say, of insistent worry about keeping a marriage together or finding a way to pay medical bills, then it inflicts serious wear and tear on both brain and body.

Wear and tear occur because stress throws the body out of balance. The human body wants at any moment to be in balance. It wants to work in ways that will provide it with precisely the right levels of things it needs to thrive, such as the right amounts of oxygen and acidity, and the necessary body temperature. When stress upsets this balance, the stressed brain says to the body, "I am under stress. Heart, beat faster. Blood, please flow mostly to the muscles. Lungs, take in more air than usual to increase your breathing rate. Hypothalamus, signal the pituitary gland to initiate steps that prompt the adrenal gland and start it producing cortisol."

Ironically, the body's attempt to overcome stress and restore balance may cause illness.[56] When the brain attempts to restore the body's balance, it initiates the secretion of hormones by means of the HPA (hypothalamic-pituitary-adrenal) pathway. Imagine that a speeding car aims straight for you just as you begin to cross the street. Stress kicks in, and immediately your brain sets in motion the HPA pathway That is, it tells the hypothalamus, located deep inside the brain, to send CRF (corticotropin releasing factor) to the pituitary gland. This CRF commands the pituitary gland to release the hormone ACTH (adrenocorticotropic hormone) into the bloodstream. The ACTH then travels to the adrenal gland. When the ACTH hits the adrenal gland, it stimulates that gland to produce, among other hormones, cortisol.

This cortisol helps the body generate the energy it needs to jump out of the way of the speeding car and reach safety. Cortisol produces this life-saving energy by entering the bloodstream and acting on various sites to speed up the heart rate, increase blood pressure, and increase the breathing rate.[57] Accelerating these functions boosts the supply of glucose—the energy—available to the brain and heart.

Once the cortisol gives muscles the energy they need to leap out of the way of the speeding car, the crisis is past and the cortisol is no longer required. It should therefore leave the system quickly and allow the body to regain its balance. If the cortisol does in fact leave the system quickly, it does no harm. However, great harm afflicts both brain and body when cortisol remains in the system for weeks and months, as happens in cases of chronic stress. Suppose that Sam, a Boeing engineer, worries that any day Boeing may lay him off. Because Sam's worry goes on for months and never diminishes, neither does the cortisol in his system. The constant presence of cortisol in Sam's body can cause a variety of problems.

For example, cortisol causes the body to send energy out to the muscles. When it does so for weeks and months, eventually the body becomes incapable of storing surplus energy. Lacking a store of surplus energy, the body suffers great fatigue. Cortisol also makes the heart pump at a heightened rate. When cortisol stays for a long time in the body, forcing the heart constantly to pump at an increased rate, the result is chronic high blood pressure leading to cardiovascular disease. Furthermore, cortisol disrupts the immune system. When cortisol remains in the body for an extended period, disrupting the immune system, the body becomes susceptible to various diseases. Cortisol also suppresses digestion, and when digestion is suppressed for weeks or months, ulceration and colitis result.[58]

Living in a condition of perpetual stress, living with high levels of cortisol, harms not only the body's functions, but also the brain. It disrupts and disorganizes brain circuits, causing a decreased branching of dendrites both in the hippocampus and in the prefrontal cortex. We have seen that these areas are vital for memory and logical thinking.[59] Stress also interferes with new cell growth in the dentate gyrus, a subsystem of the hippocampus.

Fortunately, a number of strategies help adults mitigate stress. Among the most effective antidotes to stress are confiding in a good friend, playing, meditating, becoming absorbed in a hobby, concentrating on good news, seeking occasions to laugh, and becoming mindful of reasons to be grateful.

Neuroscience has learned that stress affects not only adults, but also infants and very young children. When an infant is vaccinated, for example, stress causes the infant's body to produce cortisol. When a baby boy is circumcised, his body also generates cortisol. Babies suffer stress and produce cortisol not only when they experience pain, but also when their environment is unloving. If a caregiver is harsh, or if the caregiver is neglectful, preoccupied, and indifferent, those in her care suffer stress. Even if the caregiver in a day-care center is loving, children who must remain in day-care for many hours eventually experience stress, and their cortisol levels increase.[60]

Neuroscientists delivered sobering news when they discovered that in children, as in adults, stress disrupts the body's balance and damages both brain and body. Their discovery challenges us to shield children from stress and reduce it in our own lives.

Endnotes: Chapter Three

1. Samuel Johnson, *The Idler*, no. 44 (February 17, 1759).

2. Gerald M. Edelman, *Second Nature: Brain Science and Human Knowledge* (New Haven: Yale University Press, 2006), p. 21; Robert M. Sapolsky, *Biology and Human Behavior: The Neurological Origins of Individuality, 2nd edition,* (Chantilly, Virginia: The Teaching Company, 2005), pp. 19-37.

3. Joseph Le Doux, *The Emotional Brain* (New York: Simon & Schuster, 1996), p. 213.

4. Le Doux, *The Emotional Brain,* p. 213.

5. Antonio Damasio, *Descartes' Error* (New York: Avon Books, 1994), p. 101. See also Michael S. Sweeney, *Brain: The Complete Mind* (Washington D.C: National Geographic, 2009), p.43; The brain's circuits engage in parallel processing; information passes along parallel circuits to allow us to have a unified memory. "A single neuron may excite several others... This causes 'parallel processing' of information as circuits diverge and converge in the central nervous system. Each neural circuit delivers different information at the same time. For example, seeing a kitten may remind you of the cat you raised as a child; the scar on your hand . . .or . . . pleasant purring . . . ."

6. Rita Carter, *Mapping the Mind* (Berkeley: University of California Press, 1998), p. 160; See also Janeen Interlandi, "Mysteries of Memory," *Newsweek* (22 Sept. 2008).

7. William H. Calvin, *How Brains Think* (New York: Basic Books, 1996), p. 116.

8. On long term potentiation, see Carter, *Mapping the Mind,* pp. 159-164, 176-179; Sapolsky, *Biology and Human Behavior,* p. 19.

9. Daniel Siegel, *The Developing Mind,* (New York: The Guilford Press, 1999), pp. 28-29.

10. Damasio, *Descartes' Error,* pp. 41; 84. Italics mine.

11. Carter, *Mapping the Mind,* p. 190.

12. Damasio, *Descartes' Error,* pp. 41; 84.

13. Neil A. Campbell, Lawrence G. Mitchell, Jane B. Reece, *Biology: Concepts and Connections* (New York: Benjamin/Cummings Publishing, 1994), p. 563; Daniel L. Schacter, *Searching for Memory* (New York: Basic Books, 1996), pp. 41-43; Carter, *Mapping the Mind,* pp. 188-189.

14. Joseph LeDoux, "The Power of Emotions," in *States of Mind,* ed. Roberta Conlan (New York: Dana Press and John Wiley & Sons, Inc., 1999), pp. 146-147; see also. Schacter, pp. 42-43; Rita Carter, Susan Aldridge, Martyn Page, Steve Parker, *The Human Brain Book* (New York: DK Publishing, 2009), pp. 154-155; Carter, *Mapping the Mind,* p. 190.

15. David A. Sousa, *How the Brain Learns* (Reston, VA: NASSP, 1995), p. 18.

16. Sweeney, p. 42; John Medina, *Brain Rules* (Seattle: Pear Press, 2008), p. 105.

17. Carter, *Mapping the Mind,* pp. 160-166. For information on H.M. see Carter, pp. 169-172. Robert Sylwester, *A Celebration of Neurons* (Alexandria, VA: ASCD), 1995, p. 45; Sue Halpern, "Forgetting is the New Normal," *Your Brain: A User's Guide* (New York: Time, Inc, 2009), p. 72.

18. Damasio, *Descartes' Error,* p. 100.

19. Medina, pp. 147, 100, 110.

20. Calvin, p.2.

21. Sylwester, p. 51; Damasio, *Descartes' Error,* p. 239.

22. Benedict Carey, "How Nonsense Sharpens the Intellect," *The New York Times* (October 6, 2009), <http://www.nytimes.com/2009/10/06> downloaded 10-6-2009.

23. Michael Gazzaniga, *The Ethical Brain* (New York: Dana Press, 2005), p.148.

24. Gazzaniga, *The Ethical Brain,* p. 149; See also Michael Gazzaniga, *Human* (New York: HarperCollins, 2008), pp. 117-118.

25. Gazzaniga, *The Ethical Brain,* p. 151.

26. Gazzaniga, *The Ethical Brain,* p. 151.

27. LeDoux, *The Emotional Brain,* p. 32.

28. Siegel, p. 28: "Memory is not a static thing, but an active set of processes... Remembering is not merely the reactivation of an old engram; it is the construction of a new neural net profile with features of the old engram and elements of memory from other experiences, as well as influences form the present state of mind."

29. LeDoux, *The Emotional Brain,* p. 210.

30. Schacter, p. 43.

31. John J. Ratey, *A User's Guide to the Brain,* (New York: Vintage, 2002), p. 226. See also LeDoux, *The Emotional Brain,* pp. 23, 26.

32. LeDoux, *The Emotional Brain,* p. 23.

33. Carter, *Mapping the Mind,* pp. 82; 83; 32-47. See especially Joseph Le Doux, "The Power of Emotions," in *States of Mind,* ed. Roberta Conlan, pp. 125-126: "The brain does not have a single system dedicated to the function of 'emotion'. Instead the various classes of the mental states that we collectively refer to as emotion are mediated by separate neural systems . . . .so the subjective feelings that occur when these systems are activated . . have unique neural underpinnings . . . The brain mechanisms that generate a given mental state, or . . . emotion, also give rise to . . . physiological states, such as pulse rates . . . . Feelings, by contrast are a conscious subjective experience."

34. LeDoux, "The Power of Emotions," p. 125.

35. Ratey, pp. 225-226.

36. The Compact Edition of the Oxford English Dictionary (New York: Oxford University Press, 1971).

37. David G. Myers, "The Powers and Perils of Intuition: Understanding the Nature of Our Gut Instincts, *Scientific American Mind* (June/July, 2007), pp. 24-29.

38. LeDoux, *The Emotional Brain,* p. 25.

39. This description of structures in the limbic system relies on Jeanette Norden,

Understanding the Brain, Chantilly, VA: The Teaching Company, 2007), pp. 89-100 and John Ratey, p. 227.

40. Carter, *Mapping the Mind,* pp. 82-90; Louis Cozolino, *The Neuroscience of Human Relationships* (New York: W.W. Norton & Company, 2006), pp. 164-168. The amygdala consists of a set of large clusters of neurons that become active in response to both pleasant and negative stimuli. It appraises signals to see if they present danger, and if the amygdala feels threatened, it tells the hypothalamus to direct the autonomic nervous system to initiate the fight, flight, or freeze response.

41. The amygdala alerts the hypothalamus to release CRH, a hormone that stimulates the pituitary gland. The pituitary gland therefore releases the hormone ACTH. This hormone stimulates the adrenal glands, causing them to produce the stress hormone cortisol. Cortisol prompts the body's freeze, flight, or fight response. See MCWEN GOES HEREBruce McEwen, "Stress and the Brain," in *States of Mind,* ed. Roberta Conlan figure 6, p. 86.

42. Joseph LeDoux, "The Power of Emotions," p. 147.

43. Damasio, *Descartes'Error* , pp. 38-41.

44. Ratey, p. 231.

45. Damasio, *Descartes' Error,* pp. 43-52; Gazzaniga, *Human,* p. 120.

46. Numerous versions of the famous Trolley Problem, invented by Philippa Foot and Judith Jarvis Thomson, have been posited. Cognitive neuroscientists Joshua Greene and Jonathan Cohen took MRIs of those engaged in the Trolley Problem. They saw that when the Problem became personal, the part of the brain involved in emotion—the medial frontal lobes—competed with the dorsolateral frontal lobes that engaged in cold analysis. See on the Trolley Problem, for example, Jeffrey Kluger, "What Makes Us Moral?" *Your Brain: A User's Guide* (New York: Time, Inc., 2009), pp. 86-87; Gazzaniga. *The Ethical Brain,* pp. 155,170. A version used by Harvard scientist Joshua Greene is described by Robert Wright, "How We Make Life-and-Death Decisions," *Time* January 29, 2007, p. 116. See also Joshua Greene, "From Neural 'Is' To Moral 'Ought': What Are the Moral Implications of Neuroscientific Moral Psychology?" *Nature Reviews Neuroscience,* (2003, Vol. 4), pp. 847-850. Jonah Lehrer discussed the Trolley Problem in his lecture "How We Decide: From Brains to Behavior," OHSU Brain Awareness Lecture Series, February 1, 2010.

47. Jorge Moll and Ricardo de Oliveira-Souza, "When Morality is Hard to Like: How Do We Juggle Evidence and Emotions to Make a Moral Decision?" *Scientific American Mind* (February/March 2008), pp. 30-35.

48. Sharon Begley, "Heard Any Good Stories Lately?" *Newsweek* (September 22, 2008), p. 42.

49. Cozolino, p. 85.

50. Daniel Goleman, *Emotional Intelligence* (New York: Bantam Books, 1995), pp. 46-67.

51. Richard E. Nisbett, *Intelligence and How to Get It* (New York: W.W. Norton & Company, 2009), p. 187.

52. Humberto Maturana and Pille Bunnell, "Biosphere, Homosphere, and Robospheres: What has that to do with Business?" Paper based on a presentation made by Humberto Maturana at the Society for Organizational Learning meeting, Amherst, Massachusetts, June, 1998, <http://www.sol-ne.org/res/wp/maturana> downloaded 27 Jan. 1999. See

also, Humberta Maturana and Pille Bunnell, "The Biology of Business: Love Expands Intelligence," *Reflections,* vol. 1, number 2, pp. 10-12.

53. See Marion Diamond, Janet Hopson, *Trees of the Mind* (New York: Plume Book, 1999) p. 127; Sylwester, pp. 44-45, 88-90; Michael D. Lemonick, "The Many Flavors of Memory," *Your Brain: A User's Guide,* (New York: Time, Inc., 2009), pp. 78-81.

54. Goleman, *Emotional Intelligence,* pp. 20-22. The amygdala activates the hippocampus to give us enduring memory. See LeDoux, "The Power of Emotions," p. 142: The amygdala is a "feeling center." It gives you unconscious memory, whereas "the hippocampal system gives you conscious memory of an emotional experience." Also LeDoux, p. 141: "The amygala and hippocampus systems mediate separate kinds of memory."

55. Robert M. Sapolsky, *Why Zebras Don't Get Ulcers: an Updated Guide to Stress, Stress-Related Disease, and Coping* (New York: W. H. Freeman and Company, 1994), p. 3.

56. Sapolsky, *Why Zebras,* pp.7- 8: "The stress-response can be mobilized not only in response to physical or psychological insults, but also in expectation of them. . . .It is . . . a physiological system activated . . . by all sorts of physical disasters [and] by just thinking about them . . ." See also p. 16.

57. Sapolsky, *Why Zebras,* p. 23.

58. Sapolsky, *Why Zebras,* pp. 8-17.

59. McEwen, pp. 84-88; Sapolsky, *Why Zebras,* pp. 19-36.

60. Megan Gunnar, "Stress and the Young Child," OHSU lecture, Portland, Oregon, February 12, 2003.

CHAPTER 4

How Relationships Forge the Brain

"Love yourself, then forget it. Then, love the world."
Mary Oliver. *To Begin with, the Sweet Grass.*

"The loss of relationship, with its consequent alienation,
is a kind of supreme evil in the universe."
Brian Swimme, Thomas Berry. *The Universe Story.* 1992.

Relationships forge the Self

THIRTY YEARS AGO, THE FIELD OF *SOCIAL* NEUROSCIENCE DID not exist. Today experts in social neuroscience are probing what happens in the human brain when people interact with one another. Their findings indicate that relationships shape the unique, one-of-a-kind self that each of us calls "I."[1] From interacting with others, the brain learns to feel a shared humanity, develops empathy and compassion, learns to interpret social cues, raises intelligence, and cultivates personality traits. Who we are is not decreed by our genes. The "I," the self, gradually emerges day by day largely as a result of our relationships.[2]

At birth, many neural circuits are already connected and up and running. Circuits that enable the heart to beat, blood to circulate, and lungs to breathe are established and will not change. At birth, however, a great many neurons that have been genetically programmed to let us do specific things such as see, hear, and feel compassion will not function properly until experience joins them into circuits. As Helen Neville of the University of Oregon said, "Virtually every brain system that we know about—visual systems, auditory systems, attentional systems, language systems— is importantly shaped by experience. . . . Some brain systems are much more plastic than others. Some are plastic only during limited periods, while some are capable of change throughout life."[3]

A great part of human experience involves relating to others. We human beings are sociable through and through. Gracious relationships make our hearts sing. It is true that occasionally people enjoy solitude, but humans are designed to socialize.[4] The brain, a social organ, likes to talk, laugh, hug, play, and celebrate with other brains. In fact, the human brain not only enjoys relationships. It demands them. It requires the company of other brains because relationships sculpt the self.

How do you regard yourself? Do you feel good about yourself? Do you see yourself as capable and likable, someone worth knowing who can get the job done? Are you confident that others will find you good company? Or do you regard yourself as an inept failure, unlikable and dull?

How do you interact with others? Are you the kind of person who, when stuck in a very slow supermarket line, talks cheerfully to strangers, passing the time in a genial way, creating a brief sense of camaraderie? Or do you stand in that line feeling trapped and wishing that the clerk would stop making small talk with customers and move faster? When you meet someone for the first time, are you open, accepting, and glad to welcome a new acquaintance? Or are you hesitant and wary, thinking, "Prove yourself. I don't know you, and I'm not sure I want to."

How do you view the world? Do you look with dismay and hopeless resignation on the effects of climate change, war, unemployment, and the machinations of investment bankers? Or do you expect human beings to find enduring solutions to these problems? Relationships helped make you the way you are. Relationships influence the organization and functioning of the developing brain, and relationships continue throughout life to design the brain.

The child's most important relationship

Because young brains have great plasticity, the most important relationship a child can have is with a loving adult. John Ratey of the Harvard Medical School explains that "genes and the environment work together to shape our brains, and we can manage them both if we want to."[5] If we have the will, we can provide children with a nurturing environment in which loving relationships shape young brains.[6] The power of love is something neuroscience increasingly recognizes.

When a mother smiles at her baby, "snap," the baby's brain establishes a circuit that joins the sight of the smiling mother with the emotion of happiness.[7] Similarly, when a mother touches her baby—hugs, pats and caresses her baby—her touch generates crucial circuits in the baby's brain. Touch, the baby's first experience of the world, is as important to the infant as food, water, and oxygen.[8] The mother's embrace, for example, prompts the baby's brain to make circuits in the motor cortex. In so doing, it helps fashion the part of the brain that sends signals to the muscles and influences movement. The mother's embrace also shapes neural circuits in the parietal cortex, the part of the brain that interprets touch, pain, and pressure, and that gives us a sense of space. In addition, the mother's embrace generates neural circuits that hold feelings of safety and security.

Attentive and attuned to his daughter, the loving father satisfies her needs. When he perceives that the child is cold, he wraps her in a warm blanket. When she is hungry, he feeds her. When she is tired, he puts her to bed. When she is sad, he comforts her. This prompt and sensitive attention joins together neurons in the child's brain, forging circuits that hold feelings of emotional security.[9] "When children develop secure attachments to parents," according to Daniel Siegel of the UCLA School of Medicine, "these allow them to go out into the world to explore and develop relationships with others."[10] Feeling secure enables children to get along with others, focus on work, achieve goals, and perceive obstacles not as threats, but as exciting challenges. Feeling secure helps children learn to treat others with love, affection, kindness, and acceptance.[11] It inspires them to put aside their own needs to relieve the suffering of others. It instills in them the realization that they share with others a common humanity.[12]

When children must compete for an adult's attention, or when they are made to pass the time in front of a computer or TV screen, their brains do not fashion neural circuits in which are embedded feelings of security and affectionate regard for others. The unintentional neglect of uncomprehending parents harms a child's brain as surely as does intentional and cruel abuse.

The effects of abuse and neglect

Abused and neglected children, denied the loving attention that the brain requires, do not establish neural networks that hold feelings of love and regard for others. Negative language alone is sufficient to wire the young brain in ways that impair brain function. The brain pays three to five times more attention to cruel words than it pays to positive remarks. Cruel words diminish self-confidence and erode self-respect. Unrelenting negative criticism, mockery, derision, sarcasm, taunts, insults, disparagement, and condescending rejection join neurons into circuits that hold dark feelings and anti-social behavior.

Young people who are routinely subjected to abuse and rejection feel anxious, distracted, and unable to concentrate. Demeaned and belittled every day, typically either they withdraw or burn with a sense of outrage that drives them to seek revenge against their tormentors.[13]

Unfortunately, incidents of child abuse are not uncommon. At a 2008 conference for caregivers in Colorado, for instance, a woman said that her six-year old adopted son, whom she had raised since he was two years old, remained cold and unloving no matter how much she and her husband loved and encouraged the little boy. She said that doctors had concluded that her child was unable to love because as an infant he had suffered extensive brain damage to the frontal lobe from beatings administered by his biological mother.

The terrible effects of a maimed childhood became painfully clear when Romanian orphanages were opened to the international community. In 1966 Romania's dictator Nicolae Ceausescu decreed that until women under age 45 had given birth to five children, they would be forbidden access to birth control or abortions. Because impoverished couples could not afford to care for the unwanted children that resulted from this law, they abandoned them to orphanages. Thousands of newborns were warehoused in grim facilities where one caregiver was assigned to look after as many as twenty babies.

In 1989, after Ceausescu's fall from power, the government made scores of Romanian orphans available for adoption. People from the United States, Canada, and Western Europe visited to discover the terrible consequences of raising children without touch, love, and constant one-on-one attention. In these orphanages, children were crammed into cribs so close together that an attendant could barely squeeze between them. Tightly swathed in blankets, the children were treated like inanimate objects. They were never held, not even to be fed. Instead, a bottle was propped against the crib's railings. They were picked up only briefly, once a day, when a diaper was pulled off, used as a wipe, and replaced by another. The foul stench in the orphanage—ironically, windows were kept shut against infection—exacerbated the horrible condition of these zombie-like children who did not smile or cry.[14]

Because they were never hugged, never loved, and never given affectionate attention, these children did not learn to love. Their brains did not create circuits to hold feelings of security, shared humanity, compassion, and kindness. No one came when they cried, so they stopped crying. No one talked to the children, so they could barely speak. These children rarely set foot outside their cribs, so they had trouble walking. Anxious, living in a state of stress, they did not grow at normal rates. An eleven-year old girl, for instance, was the size of a normal four-year old. The hippocampus, temporal lobes, and frontal cortex all suffered neuronal loss, impairing the children's intellectual development and emotional stability.

A young woman from Utah told me that when she visited a Romanian orphanage to adopt a child, she placed an *m&m* candy in a two-year old's hand. No one had ever before unexpectedly put anything in that toddler's hand, certainly not candy. Having no idea what to make of this strange experience, the toddler sat immobile and stared at the candy in her open hand until the visiting woman finally removed it.

Various studies of what befell the Romanian orphans after they were adopted suggest the great power of early experiences to shape the brain. Some children who were adopted from these orphanages did manage to adapt and live normal lives. A great many, however, never recovered from the neglect they suffered as infants.[15] A substantial number of the adopted children had severe problems, including impaired IQ. Babies adopted before the age of two were able to recover about half their IQ, but those adopted after the age of two and a half had sustained too much neural loss to reclaim their intelligence.

Brain damage also made it impossible for many of these adopted children to establish normal relationships. Deprived of opportunities to develop emotionally and socially, these children found it hard to get along with their peers. They avoided other children. Withdrawn and timid, they regarded their adoptive parents and siblings with detachment. Joseph Le Doux sees "the personality disorders of children raised in brutal Romanian orphanages as a shocking testimony" to the fact that relationships have profound effects on behavior.[16] The stories of two thirteen-year old boys illustrate the power of early childhood experiences to shape the human brain.

One thirteen year old, Seth (a fictitious name) was adopted at age two. Seth never loved his adoptive parents. He cared no more for his father than he did for the barber who cut his hair, and his mother inspired no more fondness than did the lady behind the grocery story counter. Although Seth did not feel love for his adoptive parents, however, he did recognize intellectually that they were good people who treated him well. Consequently he worked hard to learn and mimic affectionate words and gestures. By the age of thirteen, Seth was, as his father explained, "getting better" at figuring out how to connect with his adoptive parents. "He still doesn't feel an emotional bond with us, but he knows when to give his mom a hug and when it's appropriate to say 'I love you.' He may not feel love, but he gets the idea of expressing fondness."

Far less fortunate were the parents of a different thirteen year old, here given the fictitious name Carl. Carl lived neglected in a Russian orphanage until he was seven years old. At the age of seven, he was adopted and began to live in the United States with his adoptive parents and their biological nine-year old daughter. At the age of thirteen, Carl killed his fifteen year old step-sister with a knife. He was not sorry, nor could he understand why he should be punished.[17] When cruel and callous adults around the world inflict suffering on children, they scar the child's brain as surely as they scar the body.

Bullying

Because relationships shape a loving brain, the gradual decline of society into a state of relational poverty should greatly concern us. Is a sense of shared humanity eroding? Could electronic communication, as it replaces face-to-face contact, be contributing to the demise of strong personal bonds? How do we relate to one another in the twenty-first century?

A telling example of growing relational poverty is the increase in bullying that has occurred over the past decade. Adults as well as young people practice, or condone, bullying. Bullying is common in schools all over the world. To condone or ignore bullying, however, is unconscionable. Bullying is *aggressive cruelty*. It is aggressive cruelty, furthermore, intentionally and repeatedly inflicted *on those perceived to be defenseless.* In elementary school, sixth graders admitted to bullying not just classmates they disliked, but even avowed friends. Fifty-six percent of all students in grades six through eight say they have cyber-bullied a friend. Middle school girls are notorious for using Twitter, text messages, e-mail and Facebook to bully their peers. By using mean, vulgar, and threatening verbal attacks, and by disclosing embarrassing private information, middle school girls seek to publicly humiliate their victims. Teenage bullies in high school also rely on cyberspace to decimate those they deem undesirable. Typically these bullies come from permissive and unstructured homes where they receive little mentoring. They lack empathy and disdain moral rules. Their fierce cyberspace assaults leave their victims disheartened and mortified.

Perhaps those adults who dismiss acts of bullying as the insignificant pranks of ebullient youth are themselves bullies. Certainly bullying does occur among adults. Doctors, lawyers, and university professors are especially inclined to be bullies. They bully, respectively, nurses, paralegals, and graduate students whose dependent positions make them vulnerable. As it happens, fifty-seven percent of the bullying that occurs in the workplace is perpetrated by women who believe, evidently, that domineering, tough leaders produce good results.[18] The story of Enron, of course, belies such a myth.

Corporate bullying at Enron

Richard D. Kinder served as president of Enron for ten years, from 1986 to 1996. These years were good for the company and good for the company's employees because Kinder understood that open, honest, respectful relationships generate a transparent organization in which employees are intrinsically motivated to excel. With this in mind, Kinder made it a point to work closely with his managers. He asked them to produce timely reports, which he studied with great care. Kinder also held regular meetings with each individual manager when he asked them detailed questions. As a result, Kinder knew exactly what his managers were doing and was familiar with everything happening throughout the company. Kinder required his managers to hold similar meetings with the employees who reported to them. This openness and candor generated an atmosphere of honesty and trust. Because Kinder paid attention to each employee, furthermore, Enron felt like family.

For instance when a manager could not afford to travel home to attend a family funeral, Kinder gave him time off and the financial means to attend.

From 1997-2001, Jeffrey Skillings served as Enron's president. Skillings was apparently oblivious of the inspiring impetus that positive relationships give to any organization. As a consequence, he destroyed the company's culture of trust and mutual respect, and, ultimately, destroyed the company itself. Behaving like a bully, Skillings made decisions based on two convictions. He believed that people are by nature greedy and therefore value money above all else. He also believed that cut-throat competition in a "survival of the fittest" atmosphere, not collaboration, motivates people to work hard and succeed.

True to his misguided convictions, Skillings set up a bonus and evaluation system that he named the "Peer Review Committee System," and that workers termed "Rank and Yank." The brutal system of evaluation reflected the premise that greed and fear drive performance. Skillings' system of "Rank and Yank" was designed to frighten and publicly humiliate—to bully—employees. "Rank and Yank" graded people on a scale of one to five, one being a good rating, five being failure. The results of an employee's formal review were actually made public on the company's Web page, along with the employee's photograph. In this way, public humiliation became institutionalized. Employees whose evaluations were riddled with mere fives were allowed two weeks to find another place at Enron. If they failed, they were fired. Ten to twenty percent of the entire workforce was fired every six months. As a result of this destructive evaluation system, employees undermined one another. People deceived and betrayed others to keep their own jobs. Honesty vanished, as did trust and candor. People practiced secrecy, fear, and brutality as they struggled to manipulate and boost their own ranking. Skillings had not learned from neuroscience the truth that Richard Kinder intuited, namely, that good relationships, far more than money, inspire human beings to feel satisfied with their lives. Cooperation is the human being's biological condition, not competition. Indeed, the survival and evolution of the human species undoubtedly depended above all on the human's capacity to be sociable and cooperate rather than compete. Cooperation and a sense of belonging, not competition, aid survival.[19]

Belonging makes us happy

We flourish above all when we belong. Belonging is a prerequisite for happiness. Human beings need so much to belong that they become attached to artificial characters in movies and bond with contestants on TV reality shows. The human desire to belong is so strong that it causes self-employed people all over the United States to pay about $350 a month to rent a desk in a common space where others also sit at their rented desks. Rather than work alone at home, they pay for the opportunity to work in a place that offers them companionship. Research suggests that more than money, positive interactions at work determine how satisfied people are with their jobs and their lives.[20]

The sociable brain needs so urgently to belong that its favorite default activity is to review its social life. When the brain is sitting around doing nothing in particular, when it is relaxing and not concentrating, it spends its down-time appraising its relationships. The brain asks, "Was I accepted? Did I say the right thing? Did they respect me? Did I belong?" The brain thinks about others all the time. When human beings are cut off from others for prolonged periods, when for whatever reason they are unable to interact with others for an extended time, they suffer and are likely to die.[21]

Social in bone, heart, and brain, we human beings use conversation as a way to belong. We especially enjoy gossip because gossiping makes us feel included. Men and women alike gossip, mainly about personal matters. Cell phone conversations are rarely about the causes of the Civil War or Plato's *Republic*. Women spend one-third of their conversation talking about themselves—their physical state, tastes, and activities: "I need to lose five pounds." "Yellow and white flowers are my favorites." "We never miss a home basketball game." Keenly interested in others, women spend two-thirds of their conversation talking about other people. "The last time I saw her, she looked exhausted." "He does all the cooking for the family, and she does the cleaning." "Ellen has dimples and a sharp tongue."

Men also love to gossip. They may call it networking or trading stories, but it is still just gossip. Unlike women, men spend not one-third, but two-thirds of their time talking about themselves: "I biked eighty miles yesterday on mountain roads." "We had seats on the fifty yard line." "I convinced the boss to adopt a new plan." Gossip helps people order and interpret their experiences at the same time that it bolsters a sense of belonging.[22]

The pain of not belonging

Belonging is so important that if we do not belong, we suffer actual pain. When we do not belong—when we feel rejected, ignored, mocked, or reprimanded—we experience the same hurt that physical pain causes. Two brain regions respond to physical pain. The same two regions also respond to social pain. These two regions are the anterior cingulate cortex, located deep inside the prefrontal cortex, and the right ventral prefrontal cortex. Both react to the pain of a broken arm, and both also react to the

"Social pain is real. . . Social distress activates the same neural circuits that physical pain activates"

Images of physical pain and social pain

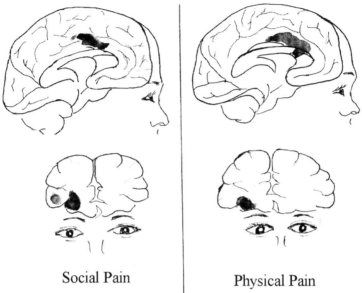

Social Pain   Physical Pain

The dorsal anterior cingulate cortex, highlighted top, indicates pain. The prefrontal cortex, bottom, shows pain being regulated. Based on illustrations by Samuel Valasco in Naomi Eisenberger, Lieberman, Williams, *Science*, 2003.

FIGURE 6

pain of social distress. When you break your arm, or when you are rejected, your anterior cingulate cortex immediately sends out an alarm: "Pain...something is terribly wrong." This alarm serves to alert the right ventral prefrontal cortex to minimize the pain as much as possible.[23] The discovery that the neural systems for physical pain also handle social pain shows that social pain is real.

The pain of not belonging is so intense that we try hard to avoid it. To avoid the pain of not belonging, for instance, we may conform,[24] repeating the same ideas and attitudes that our friends and colleagues voice. We may accept culture's dictates and willingly become prisoners of context, physical and mental.

Those who are confident that they belong, however, and who feel secure, often transcend self-interest and put others ahead of themselves. Typically it is the people who feel accepted and appreciated that strive to make sure others feel accepted, too. Instead of acting like an ego encased in skin asking always, "How am I doing? How am I doing?" people with a sense of belonging want to make sure that others also feel included.[25] Neuroscience suggests that everyone's responsibility is to include, understand, and value others. Belonging is so necessary for survival that it triggers the reward circuit.

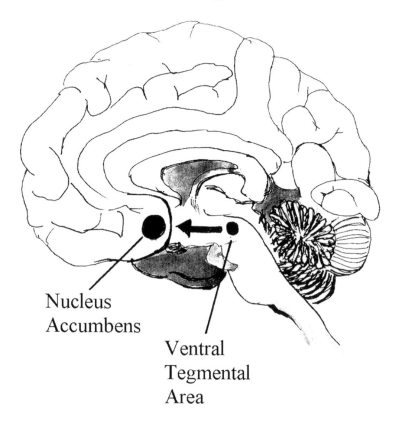

Nucleus
Accumbens

Ventral
Tegmental
Area

The Reward Circuit

FIGURE 7

The reward circuit

When we feel that we belong—that we are connected to a social group—the brain rewards us with a great sense of pleasure. Physical pleasure stimulates the reward circuit, also known as the pleasure pathway. Belonging stimulates the same reward circuit. Just as *social distress* activates the *same neural circuits that physical pain* activates, so *social pleasure* arouses the same neural circuits that *physical pleasure* activates.[26]

The brain's reward circuit is located deep in the center of the brain. When something positive happens—for example, when friends invite you to dinner—your brain experiences the mental realization that something good has happened to you. Your prefrontal cortex thinks, "This was good." At the same time that your brain thinks, "A good thing happened," you enjoy a feeling of pleasure. This feeling of pleasure is the brain's reward. Whenever you do something the brain likes, the brain gives you a pleasurable sensation. The feeling of pleasure that you feel when you hear encouragement from a colleague, enjoy a picnic, or eat ice cream is the brain's bonus.

Imagine that on a hot summer day you sip a cool drink. Immediately neural circuits send a sensory stimulus that gives the cortex the mental realization that something good has happened. Once the cortex gets this sensory signal, it sends its own signal to the ventral tegmental area, a tiny little group of neurons—a one inch strip of tissue—in the mid-brain, the very center of the brain (between the brain stem and the forebrain). The ventral tegmental area's job is to notice how well various human needs are being satisfied. It is helped to do this by a steady flow of information from several brain regions that advise it of how well the brain's needs are being met.

When it learns of a pleasurable event, the tiny ventral tegmental area sends dopamine, which in this context acts as a pleasure neurotransmitter, to the nucleus accumbens by means of its dopamine-carrying axons. These axons travel to the nucleus accumbens, the reward center, and deliver dopamine to its dendrites. The ventral tegmental area also sends dopamine to the amygdala and hippocampus. The amygdala imparts agreeable emotions; the hippocampus preserves the memory associated with these emotions.[27] As soon as the nucleus accumbens, the reward center of the brain, receives this infusion of dopamine, it communicates with motor and emotional systems as well as with the prefrontal cortex. These areas cooperate to generate a sense of well-being.[28] Pleasure rewards you.

The brain's reward system is a powerful motivator. We like the reward feeling; liking it makes us want it again. Wanting that reward feeling again motivates us to strive hard to achieve it. This intrinsic motivation is far more effective than extrinsic motivation. Work inspired by a personal desire to excel leads to dedication and private satisfaction in a job well done. External rewards, however, condition people, especially children, to work for, and be dependent on, the approval of others. They make children vulnerable to manipulation by outside agents.

Mirror neurons

The power of relationships to refashion and change the brain has been clarified by one of the most important discoveries neuroscience has made in the last fifteen years, namely, that the brain contains a special set of neurons called *mirror neurons*. Mirror neurons intensify the brain's responsiveness to its environment. They are a special kind of neuron that makes it possible for human beings to learn and perceive by imitating others. Mirror neurons are involved "in the learning of manual skills, . . . spoken language, group cohesion, and empathy."[29]

The term "mirror neuron" was coined by Giacomo Rizzolatti,

Vittorio Gallese, and Leonardo Fogassi of the University of Parma in Italy. Rizzolatti and his colleagues at the University of Parma set forth their discovery of mirror neurons in a series of papers published in 1996. The discovery was serendipitous. The scientists were studying how individual neurons in the motor cortex of monkeys fired when the monkeys picked up different objects. One day a scientist reached out and picked up a piece of food. He noticed that as the monkeys watched him, their motor neurons fired in precisely the same way that they had fired when the monkeys themselves picked up the food. As Rizzolatti, Gallese, and Fogassi explain, "we realized that the pattern of neural activity associated with the observed action was a true representation in the brain of the act itself, regardless of who was performing it."[30] Just watching the scientist pick up food caused the monkeys' neurons to fire as they had fired when they themselves picked up nuts or raisins.[31] Because the monkeys' neurons became active not only when they reached for and picked up food, but also when they observed their trainer perform the identical action, Rizzolatti and his colleagues called these neurons *mirror neurons*. These neurons mentally mirrored the action they watched.[32]

Eventually research confirmed that mirror neurons are peppered throughout important regions on both sides of the human brain. They occur in the premotor cortex, the inferior and posterior parietal lobes, and the superior temporal sulcus, areas associated with movement, perception, interpreting feelings, discerning intentions, language, pain, and empathy. Mirror neurons are also located in the insula, a system that fires when we feel disgust. They lie in places "where multiple networks of visual, motor, and emotional processing converge."[33] Location allows these neurons to mirror, or imitate, the actions and feelings we humans observe in others.

Mirror neurons look like other neurons, but they have a surprising and unique double function. According to Rizzolatti,

Fogassi, and Gallese, "Much as circuits of neurons are believed to store specific memories within the brain, sets of mirror neurons appear to encode templates for specific actions."[34] These neurons fire both when *you do something*—that is, when you perform an action or feel an emotion, and when *you watch someone else do something*—when you watch someone else perform an action or feel an emotion. Mirror neurons cause you to perform—to imitate—in your brain the action or feeling you observe.

For example, when you watch a girl kick a soccer ball, your brain kicks the ball. When you simply listen to a description of the girl kicking the soccer ball, your mirror neurons connect to kick the ball. If you play soccer, your mirror neurons will fire more powerfully when you observe a player kick a ball than they would if you were ignorant of the game. In the same way, "the neurons in a piano player's brain fire more strongly when he is watching another person play Chopin than do the neurons of another observer with no musical training."[35] If you are an accomplished skier who watches someone else ski down the slope, your mirror neurons will fire more strongly than those of an observer who has never done downhill skiing.[36] Practice, in other words, readies mirror neurons to draw forth your potential.

Consider what happens when you see someone else feel an emotion. Your mirror neurons instantly cause your brain to mimic that same emotion. A woman smiles in happiness, and your mirror neurons cause you to feel that same happiness. Because of mirror neurons, you do not need to reason about the meaning of the woman's smile. You do not have to think to yourself, "The woman's smile makes her look happy, therefore she must be happy." Instead you instantly feel her happiness. Your mirror neurons make circuits that hold the feeling of happiness so that you experience the woman's happiness. When you see an emotion on another's face, you at once have that same feeling within yourself.

Now imagine that a friend is anxious. As you watch your friend feeling anxious, your mirror neurons wire your brain to imitate your friend's emotion. You "catch" his anxiety. His anxiety becomes yours. Now you feel anxious, too. Your anxiety triggers your amygdala to signal the hypothalamus to cause your own body to react. Your anxiety, which you caught second-hand by observing a friend's anxiety, now affects you physically as well as emotionally.[37] In the same way, laughter unites people in a moment of shared comfort and delight.

Mirror neurons, because they imitate what they see others do and feel, facilitate learning and insight. They help us learn to sit, walk, and dance. They help us learn to utter words, and they make it possible to discern another person's intentions instantly, without thinking. If Jason picks up a baseball bat and hurries towards a group of people, mirror neurons signal whether Jason's intent is to play baseball or start a fight. They also let us share an Olympic swimmer's thrill of victory.

The unique characteristics of mirror neurons suggest a biological explanation for our capacity to feel empathy—to know exactly what it is like to be another person, standing in that person's shoes. Empathy feeds compassion, and together empathy and compassion unite human beings. They transform many into one.

Each of us probably thinks of the "I" as a self-sufficient, independent person. In reality, of course, everyone is dependent in some way on others. We rely on relationships of every imaginable kind, and mirror neurons enable us to form these relationships. As V. S. Ramachandran says, "Mirror neurons were crucial in the development of the elaborate social skills, social networks and knowledge infrastructure we call culture."[38] Thanks to mirror neurons, human beings see with another's eyes, feel with another's heart, cooperate, collaborate and bond with one another. Giacomo Rizzolatti observed, "We are exquisitely social creatures.

Our survival depends on understanding the actions, intentions and emotions of others. . . . Mirror neurons allow us to grasp the minds of others not through conceptual reasoning but through direct simulation."[39]

The discovery of mirror neurons makes it clear that our actions and emotions influence others, and that others exert an equally powerful influence on us. Because of mirror neurons, whenever children watch an adult's behavior, the children "catch" that behavior. They perform in their own brains the things adults do and the feelings that adults manifest. Surely we adults must take care, then, that our behavior is worthy of emulation. We must also think carefully about what we choose to observe ourselves, and what we invite children to observe. When we human beings observe the actions and feelings of others, especially for a sustained period, our brains perform those same actions and feelings. What behavior do we want our brains to replicate?

Chapter 4: Endnotes

1. Daniel Siegel, *The Developing Mind* (New York: The Guilford Press, 1999), p. 1.

2. Daniel Goleman. *Social Intelligence* (New York: Bantam Books, 2006), pp. 40-55; Daniel Goleman, "Social Intelligence and the Biology of Leadership," *Harvard Business Review* (September, 2008), p. 74, defines the new field of social neuroscience: "Social Neuroscience—the study of what happens in the brain while people interact." See also Matthew D. Lieberman, "Social Cognitive Neuroscience," in R.F. Baumeister & K. D. Vohs, eds., *Encyclopedia of Social Psychology* (Thousand Oaks, California: Sage Press, 2007). Daniel Siegel points out in *The Mindful Brain* (New York: W. W. Norton & Co., 2007), p. 117, that certain brain structures are "crucial for emotional and social functioning." Specifically: the anterior cingulate cortex, orbital frontal cortex, and medial prefrontal cortex "enable awareness of one's own and others' mental processes," and regulate emotional responses.

3. Helen Neville, cited in Sharon Begley, *Train Your Mind, Change Your Brain* (New York: Ballantine Books, 2007), p. 75.

4. Louis Cozolino, *The Neuroscience of Human Relationships: Attachment and the Developing Social Brain* (New York: W.W. Norton & Company, Inc., 2006), p. 85.

5. John J. Ratey, *A User's Guide to the Brain* (New York: Vintage Books, 2002), p. 34.

6. John T. Cacioppo and William Patrick, *Loneliness: Human Nature and the Need for Social Connection* (New York: W.W. Norton & Co, 2008), pp.131-134. The work of Jerome Kagan, developmental psychologist at Harvard, shows that genes do not fix temperament irrevocably. On the contrary, environment acts on temperament to influence the person that the child becomes. See Daniel Goleman on Kagan *in Emotional Intelligence*(New York: Bantam Book, 1995), pp. 215-224.

7. Cozolino, pp. 84-85.

8. Cozolino, p. 103. See also John T. Cacioppo and William Patrick, *Loneliness*, pp. 129-130 for a discussion of the importance of touch to mammals as shown in an infamous experiment conducted in 1958 by Harry Harlow of the University of Wisconsin. Harlow made two surrogate mothers for infant rhesus monkeys, one made merely of wire, but with a milk bottle on it, one made of terry cloth. The monkeys preferred the surrogate that offered the soft touch of terry cloth to the wire surrogate. They went to the wire "mother" only when they were eager for milk, and they stayed only long enough to drink the milk. On attachment see also Thomas Lewis, Fari Amini, Richard Lannon, *A General Theory of Love* (New York: Vintage, 2000), p. 70.

9. Sharon Begley, *Train Your Mind, Change Your Brain* (New York: Ballantine Books, 2007), pp. 11, 170-74.

10. Daniel Siegel, *The Developing Mind* (New York: The Guilford Press, 1999), p. 71.

11. Begley, *Train Your Mind*, p. 11.

12. Begley, *Train Your Mind*, pp. 187-197.

13. "People notice the negative more than the positive," Michael Widerman, "Why It's So Hard to Be Happy," *Scientific American Mind* (February/March 2007), pp. 39; Marion Diamond and Janet Hopson, *Magic Trees of the Mind* (New York: Plume, 1999), p. 128. The human's quick reaction to threatening situations causes people to detect negative emotions in others more readily than positive emotions. Typically, we pick angry faces out of a crowd faster than happy faces.

14. Begley, *Train Your Mind* pp. 160-161. See on the effects of Romanian orphanages Marion Diamond and Janet Hopson, p. 128; John T. Cacioppo and William Patrick, *Loneliness*, pp.130-131; Rita Carter. *Mapping the Mind* (Berkeley: University of California Press, 1998), p. 91.

15. Especially during the first two years of life, loving adults affect a child's development of language, IQ, emotional balance, and social adjustment. See Elizabeth Gudrais, "The Developing Child," *Harvard Magazine* (April, 2009), pp. 34; 38-41. Charles A. Nelson III of Children's Hospital, Boston, found this to be the case when he studied a cohort of children raised in orphanages.

16. Joseph Le Doux, *The Synaptic Self* (New York: Viking, 2002), p. 5.

17. "Seth's" adoptive father discussed his son's progress after a lecture I gave in Seattle. A friend of Carl's family described this event to a large audience at one of my Boston lectures.

18. See the "U. S. Workplace Bullying Survey" by the polling firm Zogby International. 7,740 million on-line interviews showed that 57% of workplace bullying is done by women. See also the Workplace Bullying Institute, Bellingham, Washington for information about bullying.

19. Michael Shermer, "Don't Be Evil: Enron, Google and the Evolutionary Pscychology of Corporate Environment," *Scientific American Mind* (February/March, 2008), pp. 59-65.

20. Kiera Butler, "Works Well with Others," *Mother Jones* (January/ February 2008), pp. 66-69.

21. Goleman, *Social Intelligence*, p. 68.

22. Michael Gazzaniga, *Human* New York: Harper Collins, 2008), pp. 94-97.

23. Daniel Goleman, *Social Intelligence*, pp. 112-114. Matthew Lieberman and Naomi Eisenberger, working at UCLA, discovered that the anterior cingulate cortex acts as a neural alarm system when a person experiences social distress and alerts other parts of the brain to react appropriately. Carter, *Mapping the Mind*, p. 114, notes that pain affects the anterior cingulate cortex. This structure makes us aware of both physical and social pain. Social distress over being ostracized or unfairly treated triggers the anterior cingulate cortex. This structure integrates input from the entire cortex with the limbic system. Located deep inside the prefrontal cortex, the anterior cingulate cortex is activated by physical and social pain. The anterior cingulate cortex, the seat of dynamic vigilance, is active when we have pain or social stress. See Elkhonon Goldberg, *The Executive Brain* (New York: Oxford University Press, 2001), pp. 142-143.

Emotional pain is comparable to physical pain. See Naomi I. Eisenberger and Matthew D. Lieberman, "Why it hurts to be left out: The neurocognitive overlap between physical and social pain," *Trends in Cognitive Sciences*(2004) vol. 8, pp. 294-300; "Scientists Find Connections in the Brain Between Physical and Emotional Pain," *JAMA* (November 12, 2003), vol. 290. no. 18; David Rock, "Managing with the Brain in Mind," *Strategy+Business*, issue 56, pp. 59-65; Gazzaniga, *Human*, pp. 168 -173.

Status affects belonging: see Michael Marmot, *The Status Syndrome* (New York: Holt Paperbacks, 2004), pp. 16-43.

24. On conforming see Ervin Laszlo, *The Systems View of the World* (New York: George Braziller, 1972), p. 44.

25. Michael Gazzaniga, *Human*, pp. 94-97; 168 -173.

26. Matthew D. Lieberman and Naomi I. Eisenberger, "Pains and Pleasures of Social Life," *Science* (13 February 2009), , vol 323, pp. 890-891.downloaded from www.sciencemag.org; M. D. Lieberman, "Social Cognitive Neuroscience," in R. F. Baumeister and K. D. Vohs, eds, *Encyclopedia of Social Psychology.* (Thousand Oaks, CA: Sage Press, 2007).

27. The reward system also delivers acetylcholine, which helps consolidate new circuits. Acetylcholine helps the brain pay attention and sharpen memories, thus aiding learning and remembering. The reward center is involved in addiction. Liking the reward feeling makes us want it again. An unhealthy pleasure—like addiction to heroine—creates a wanting that is unrestrained. Eventually addicts seek a drug not to obtain pleasure, but to keep the user from experiencing the pain of withdrawal.

The process of passing on pleasure stops with re-uptake. Dopamine, having been delivered from the axon to receptors, is then released from the receptors and is pumped back into the axon of the neuron that released it to begin with. Excess dopamine is taken back up by the sending neuron. To eliminate excess dopamine, furthermore, other nerve cells release GABA, an inhibitory neurotransmitter that prevents the receiving neuron from becoming over stimulated. However, addictive drugs prevent re-uptake—that is, they prevent the re-absorption of excess dopamine. And they block the production of GABA. The normal production of neurotransmitters is badly disrupted.

28. On the reward system see Rita Carter, Susan Aldridge, Martyn Page, Steve Parker, *The Human Brain Book* (London: DK, 2009), p. 128; Jerrold S. Meyer, Linda F. Quenzer, *Psychopharmacology: Drugs, the Brain and Behavior* (Sunderland, Massachusetts: Sinazier Assoc., Inc: 2005), p. 125; Michael S. Sweeney, *Brain: The Complete Mind* (Washington DC: National Geographic, 2009), pp. 47-49; Kelley Lambert, "Depressingly Easy" *Scientific American Mind* (August/September 2008), pp. 34-35. A succinct explanation of the reward system is available in Silvia Helena Cardoso, "Hardwired for Happiness," The Dana Foundation, December 15, 2006: "When the cortex has received and processed a sensory stimulus indicting a reward, it sends a signal to the ventral tegmental area (VTA) in the midbrain. The VTA then releases dopamine not only into the nucleus accumbens, but also into the septum, the amygdala and the prefrontal cortex." <http://www.dana.org/printerfriendly.aspx.id=5514>

29. Cozolino, p. 187.

30. Giacomo Rizzolatti, Leonardo Fogassi, Vittorio Gallese, "Mirrors in the Mind," *Scientific American* (November, 2006), p. 56.

31. J. Madeleine Nash, "The Gift of Mimicry: Why Monkeys See and Do, Why Babies Smile at Mothers, and Why Our Skin Crawls at Scary Movies," *Time* (January 29, 2007), pp. 109-101; David Dobbs, Daniel Goleman and Richard Boyatzis, "Social Intelligence and the Biology of Leadership," *Harvard Business Review* (September, 2008), pp. 74-81.

32. David Dobbs, Daniel Goleman and Richard Boyatzis, "Social Intelligence and the Biology of Leadership," *Harvard Business Review* (September, 2008), pp. 24-25.

33. Cozolino, p. 187.

34. Giacomo Rizzolatti, Leonardo Fogassi, Vittorio Gallese, "Mirrors in the Mind," *Scientific American* (November, 2006), p. 56.

35. Sweeney, p. 157.

36. Sweeney, pp.156-158.

37. See Giacomo Rizzolatti, Leonardo Fogassi, Vittorio Gallese, "Mirrors in the Mind," *Scientific American* (November, 2006), pp. 54-69; David Dobbs, "A Revealing Reflection," *Scientific American Mind* (Aril/May, 2006), pp. 22-27; Louis Cozolino, pp. 186-204; J. Madeleine Nash, pp. 109-111.

38. Dobbs, cites Ramachandran, p. 27.

39. Rizzolatti cited by Sandra Blakeslee, "Cells that Read Minds," *The New York Times*, (January 10, 2006) <www.nytimes.com>, cited January 10, 2006.

CHAPTER 5

Fashioning the Moral Brain

"Between believing a thing and thinking you *know*
it is only a small step and quickly taken."
Mark Twain. *Three Thousand Years Among the Microbes.* 1905.

IT IS COMMON KNOWLEDGE THAT EACH OF US NEEDS FRIENDS, appreciates civility and courtesy, values compassion, embraces kindness, and seeks a lifetime of positive relationships. Why, then, are we so hard on one another? Ingrained habits of thought often decide how we treat others, habits that influence our moral judgments about right and wrong. The connection between habits of thought, morality, and relationships is most easily approached by considering what I call the *"H" Factor.*

The *"H" Factor*

Children learn the block letter "H" in kindergarten, or even preschool. They are drilled to recognize and print the block letter "H." Repeatedly they encounter "H" until eventually it is woven into their neurons. Eventually incoming sensations generate neural connections that contain block letter "H." Once the young brain's neural circuits hold this neural pattern, the brain is prepared, "framed," to see "H." The brain will now detect block letter "H" even when that letter occurs in grandfather's shaky, almost illegible handwriting, or in an ornate bit of calligraphy.

In the same way that the brain wires "H," so it wires the word *the*. Repeated use of *the* prepares the brain to expect to see *the*. Because our brain expects to see *the* in certain contexts, therefore we often fail to catch the error "teh" when we proofread. It is hard to catch that mistake because we are wired to see, "framed" to see, we expect to see, *the*.[1] What the brain has learned colors what it sees.

Just as frequent exposure to "H" and "the" causes the brain to shape circuits to hold "H" and "the," so frequent exposure to beliefs causes the brain to develop neural circuits that contain these specific beliefs. Once embedded in the brain, our abstract beliefs "frame"—they decide—the things we think are true or right. Wired with particular beliefs, this wiring—these neural circuits—dispose us to think what we have always thought, "see more of what we have already seen, hear anew what we have heard most often . . . ."[2] The beliefs become habitual.

Moral beliefs: universal and local

The human brain excels at generating circuits that hold habitual beliefs about right and wrong. This is because, as psychologist Steven Pinker of Harvard University puts it, a "moral sense is rooted in the design of the human brain."[3] We are born ready to be moral. From birth, genes dispose our brains to make moral distinctions. From birth, the brain is hardwired—prepared by genes—to judge human actions as either right or wrong, moral or immoral. Specific clusters of neurons let us make automatic moral judgments. Paul Bloom and his colleagues at Yale University's Infant Cognition Center have explored the moral life of babies to find that "humans do have a rudimentary moral

"We are born ready to be moral."

sense from the very start of life." Babies are not blank slates. One-year olds have a sense of right and wrong, a "general appreciation of good and bad behavior." Furthermore they want good acts to be rewarded and bad acts to be punished.

People all over the globe, according to Bloom, share a few basic concepts of right and wrong. Everywhere humans value "fairness, loyalty, kindness, [and]...deplore cruelty...."[4] Like Bloom, professors Marc Hauser and Jonathan Haidt have concluded from their respective research that humans share certain moral impulses. Hauser and Haidt, working independently, suggest that the world's cultures share some basic moral themes, or rules.[5] Although differing in small points, these scholars essentially hold that at birth the human brain is equipped with neural circuits that call for adherence to the following moral rules.

1. *Do no harm.* This rule explicitly forbids inflicting pain and suffering. By implication it requires that we help others, alleviate suffering, and oppose cruelty. It calls for compassion and empathy. Empathy is the understanding that your pain is like mine, that we are the same.[6]

The innate human desire to ease another's suffering and to avoid inflicting suffering is apparent in very young children. Studies show that toddlers try to help those who seem distressed, and preschoolers agree that hitting another person is wrong.[7]

The innate rejection of behavior that harms is not, however, uniquely human. In 1996 the story of the compassionate gorilla Binta Jua reverberated in the news. Binta Jua saved a three year old boy who fell into her zoo enclosure. The gorilla rocked the child in her arms and then carried the boy to the door and gave him to trainers.

Equally compassionate was the behavior of six rhesus monkeys who refused to inflict pain on a new addition to their group. The six monkeys had been trained to get food by pulling on a chain.

Once they knew that pulling on a chain would deliver food, their trainers introduced a seventh monkey. The newcomer got a painful shock whenever one of the six monkeys pulled a chain for food. Once the rhesus monkeys understood that pulling on the chain to get food inflicted pain on the seventh monkey, they changed their behavior to avoid hurting the newcomer. The monkeys learned that if they pulled on a different chain that delivered less food, they would not hurt the seventh monkey. Four chose to use this chain, settling for less food to spare the seventh monkey. The fifth and sixth monkeys, however, refused to pull any chain at all. They starved themselves for five and twelve days respectively to avoid shocking the seventh monkey.[8]

2. *Be fair.* Living morally demands fairness. Fairness requires reciprocation; we must return like for like. Fairness asks, for example, that we repay the kindnesses of others, reward benefactors, return favors, and punish wrongdoers. A sense of fairness asks that we practice such virtues as justice, trustworthiness, and patience.[9] A spirit of reciprocity and fairness discourages corporate corruption as surely as it discourages children from cutting into a long cafeteria line.[10]

3. *Support the community.* Human beings cannot thrive in isolation from each other. As biologist Lynn Margulis noted, although independence is merely a political conviction, interdependence is a biological condition necessary for survival. We flourish in communities. Life is a cooperative venture. Understandably, then, over time the brain developed circuitry that values the community. Virtues that strengthen the community, such as loyalty, trust, respect, and courage, we admire wholeheartedly. Similarly we admire treating others as equal in value to ourselves, self-sacrifice, and generosity because these attributes unite and preserve the community.[11] Typically we deplore as immoral any behavior that threatens the

community. Hedge fund operators, for instance, are immoral should they put personal greed ahead of the economy's health.

4. *Respect legitimate authority.* Part of the universal moral code shared by humanity calls for respecting authority. The human brain is wired to respect hierarchy and honor legitimate leaders. Respect for authority is evident, ironically, even in the operation of the countless egalitarian groups to which Americans belong. Although these groups are ostensibly egalitarian, invariably they have leaders. To that extent, they are hierarchical. The basketball team has a captain, the reading club has a chair-person, and the university has a president. Captains, chair-persons, and university presidents all rank higher than others in their group. These leaders enjoy special status. For that reason, members of their group respect them. Deference to a leader potentially benefits the community by building collegiality, minimizing conflict, generating harmony, and thus making the community cohesive.[12]

5. *Be pure:* "Purity has its roots in defending against disease: bacteria, fungi, and parasites."[13] Impurity is equated today not only with disease, but also with various other kinds of contamination. Virtually all societies reject incest, for instance, and many cultures regard disfigurement, filthy clothes, and carnality as forms of impurity. Impurity generates disgust, an emotion unique to humans.

Evidently at birth virtually all human beings possess neural circuitry, hardwiring, that disposes them to comply with these five universal moral principles, namely, to do no harm, be fair, support the community, respect legitimate authority, and be pure. Prompted from birth to adhere to these moral rules, one might expect all humans to get along together in a spirit of amicable agreement and peace.

Culture shapes morals

The problem is that interpretations of these broad moral rules differ greatly. Genes dispose us to distinguish between right and wrong. Experience, however, wires our brains with specific beliefs about what is right and what is wrong.[14] Eager to belong and equipped with mirror neurons that help us mimic what we observe, we readily assimilate local ideas, customs, practices, and values. We adopt the point of view of our family, friends, teams, clubs, and neighbors. These various social contexts assign meaning to experiences, decree rules of behavior, and issue opinions about every imaginable subject from education, politics, off-shore drilling, and the war in Afghanistan to questions about right and wrong. In this way, local culture wires our brains.

Local culture provides us with myriad contexts—work, school, church, teams—and each of these contexts prompts neurons to weave together and connect, forming the "Self." The context of one's workplace, for example, consists of physical objects (like desks, windows, and carpets), events (like attending meetings and performing specific tasks), and people (colleagues who interact, use skills, and make choices). Woven together, these objects, events, and people combine to influence the "I" that each employee calls "Self," with its convictions and morality. The groups we inhabit, the contexts we experience—culture—builds the brain continuously, moment by moment, producing our Self, the "User's Guide to the Brain." In other words, daily life builds the brain, continuously, moment by moment.

Certainly the word "culture" is often used to refer to the social inventions of people inhabiting a broad geographical region. As we have seen, however, "culture" also refers to narrow contexts such as ballet companies and NASCAR races. Economics, for example, is an academic discipline with its own culture. This academic discipline's culture does not train economists to be ethicists who ask, "How can the economy be made to serve society?" Nor does the culture of economics departments train economists to be historians disposed to ask, for instance, "Should the Federal Reserve System, created in 1913 as an entity privately owned by the nation's leading banks, continue to exist in its present form and continue to issue all U.S currency, so that the federal government must borrow money from the Federal Reserve Bank to meet its financial obligations?"

Rather than consult history, economics departments focus on designing theories, abstract models divorced from ethical and historical contexts. Their models deal with describing, analyzing, and preserving the current economy, which, for better or worse, depends on market activity leading to continuous growth. The product of a narrow culture, the economist sees through a special lens. So do we all.[15] Each of us perceives reality through the lens of our customized brain.

The brain protects the lessons of culture, the beliefs and practices it has long known, in large part because it welcomes familiar patterns that hold meaning. It resists anything that disrupts established, meaning-filled patterns.

Given that we receive our explicit ideas of right and wrong from our local community, how can we be sure that they are credible? How can we be confident that a particular deed is moral or immoral, particularly considering that morality changes as culture changes. Take, for instance, the mandate to "Be Pure." In the 1940s, smoking was acceptable. Camel cigarette commercials boasted that more doctors smoked Camels than any other cigarette. A mellifluous radio voice declared, "LSMFT—Lucky Strike Means Fine Tobacco." Advertisements promised that fine tobacco was good for the throat's "T-Zone." With time and new information, attitudes change. Today, smoking is linked with cancer, and smokers are seen increasingly in the United States as impure people doing something that is not only unhealthy, but also morally wrong. "Be pure, stop smoking." In some cultures, "be pure" forbids eating with the left hand. In some cultures the injunction "be pure" forbids women to make eye-contact with men.

This local nature of morality raises problems. Born with an innate desire to do no harm, be fair, support community, respect legitimate authority, and be pure, people do not agree, unfortunately, on the meaning of these imperatives. Nonetheless, people frequently act as if their values were definitive truths. They do so because beliefs are embedded in their neural circuits and are favored by the pattern-weaving brain as it seeks to give order and meaning to experience. In other words, our beliefs are part of us, in the same way that an arm is part of us. And just as we refuse to part with an arm and will fight to protect it, so most of us are unwilling to part with our moral convictions and will fight to protect them. People boast that they are "willing to die for their convictions."

What if these convictions, however, are easily disproved with sound evidence? What if our emotional attachment to certain beliefs defies reason? That could well be the case, given the proclivity of emotion to ignore or silence reason.

Emotion often catapults us to settle on a belief before our reason examines it. We simply *feel* that our belief is right. We embrace it emotionally. Having decided, "I like it," only then do we search for reasoned arguments and hard evidence to justify the belief. In fact, we are so determined to retain a favored belief that we intentionally push aside solid evidence showing that the belief is actually mistaken. The emotional brain "wants victory, not truth."[16] The brain wants to defend the emotionally satisfying opinion, act, or moral position that it likes so well, even if doing so tramples the facts.

To overcome the brain's narrow attachment to long-held convictions and opinions, it is necessary to approach the immediate moment thoughtfully and objectively. Only an open mind lets us circumvent the constraints of our culture-laden views. Surely a fundamental human responsibility is to see with the eyes of one who is fully aware.

Seeing, however, is not easy because *believing is seeing*.[17] The beliefs that we hold about right and wrong limit what we are willing, and therefore able, to see, hear, or understand. Overcoming beliefs that are embedded in our neural networks and that "frame" our view of friends, acquaintances, religion, politics, and everything else requires breaking habits of thought. To overcome deeply held habitual beliefs is exceptionally difficult. Habits are hard to break.

The basal ganglia: the brain's habit center

According to Ann Graybiel, the Rosenblith Professor of Neuroscience at MIT, the formation of habits takes place in the basal ganglia. *Basal ganglia* is the collective name for clusters of interconnected neurons—the caudate nucleus, putamen, globus pallidus, and substantia nigra—that communicate with each other and with some cortical regions. These clusters serve, in effect, as the brain's "habit center." An authority on the basal ganglia, Graybiel notes that its formation of habits profoundly influences the life we live.[18]

Neuroscientists realized long ago that the basal ganglia affects motor control. Deterioration of neurons in the basal ganglia is responsible for the tremors, muscle rigidity, loss of balance, and difficulties initiating and executing movement that are symptoms of Parkinson's disease.[19] Only recently, however, have scientists discovered that in addition to contributing to affecting movement, the basal ganglia is involved in the formation of habits.

Apparently the brain is always trying to automate things, turning them into habits.[20] When an activity is practiced so often that it becomes habitual—such as pulling weeds out of the garden but leaving flowers—then that activity is transferred from the cortex, where the brain thinks carefully to distinguish between weeds and flowers, to circuits in the basal ganglia. Once the process of separating weeds from flowers shifts to circuits in the basal ganglia, it becomes an established habit. Therefore it can be done automatically, leaving the thinking parts of the brain free to take up other matters. Similarly, jogging every day for several weeks triggers neural networks in the basal ganglia that make jogging habitual.

Evidently not only can actions become habitual, but so can thoughts. Just as jogging triggers neural networks that hold the habit of jogging, so thinking can trigger neurons to fire together and form circuits deep within the basal ganglia. The prefrontal cortex transmits thoughts to the subcortical structures that constitute the basal ganglia. Circuits then form in the basal ganglia to hold these "patterns of deeply held thoughts."[21] If you can recite the alphabet without thinking, or automatically spell "chameleon," evidently you can do so partly because this information has been shifted to the basal ganglia. If you can recite the multiplication tables without thinking about them, you can do so mainly because neurons in the basal ganglia wired together to hold the multiplication tables. Thus they made multiplication a habit.

Perhaps as a child you were always treated kindly and were taught to be kind to others. You valued kindness and made a point of performing kind acts. Your sustained practice throughout childhood of thinking kind thoughts and doing kind deeds wired kindness into your brain. Eventually circuitry holding kindness became embedded in your basal ganglia. Thereafter you were kind automatically, without even thinking about it.[22]

We are fortunate that the brain stores habits. We need to be able, unthinkingly, automatically, to do some things, such as multiply numbers or close a window. Automatic behavior frees the thinking parts of the brain to concentrate elsewhere.

Some habits that are wired into the brain, including the basal ganglia, may create, however, serious problems. For example, you may have the habit of eating six candy bars every day despite medical evidence that consuming excessive amounts of sugar causes illness. Although good health depends on getting rid of this destructive habit, overcoming habits is, unfortunately, extremely difficult.

It is hard to break habits partly because they produce physical changes in the brain. Alvaro Pascual-Leone, a pioneer in the study of brain plasticity, likens habits to mental "tracks" that we lay down. Once these neural tracks are in place, they become so fast and efficient that it's hard to resist them. Each time you repeat a habit, it deepens the track;[23] it strengthens the circuit. This circuitry usurps real estate in the brain; it takes over space as the habit becomes entrenched.

It is also hard to get rid of habits because they are, of course, familiar, and their very familiarity gives the brain such feelings of security, safety, and pleasure that it wants to hold them fast.[24]

Another reason that habits are hard to break is that the brain's orbital frontal cortex, its error detector, prefers keeping them.

The orbital frontal cortex: error detector

Located slightly above and behind the eyes, the orbital frontal cortex is part of the prefrontal cortex, the site of higher order thinking. Tucked into the underside of the prefrontal cortex, at the very front of the brain, the orbital frontal cortex serves as the brain's error detector. It appraises a situation to see how things are going. If it notices that something is wrong, it shouts "Mistake!" Suppose that on your way home from work you have for twenty years caught the same bus at the same time to ride up the same hill. One day the bus fails to come. You wait and wait, and still no bus. Because your expectation is broken, your orbital frontal cortex warns, "Something is wrong." Or suppose that you are driving down the highway when suddenly the car's windshield cracks. You expected the windshield to remain intact, but instead something different happened. Perhaps you expected iced tea and received lemon juice. These disappointed expectations set off the orbital frontal cortex, the brain's error detector. In the same way, expectation is thwarted when one expects to follow a habit and is prevented from doing so.

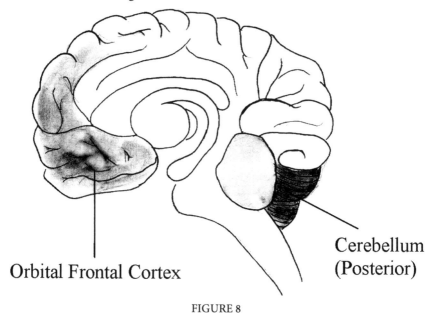

Orbital Frontal Cortex

Cerebellum (Posterior)

FIGURE 8

When someone tries to break a habit, the orbital frontal cortex detects an error. It announces that attempting to break this habit is a serious mistake. The orbital frontal cortex alerts the brain by insisting *something is wrong; something is not right!* This error alert is like a flashing orange hand at a crosswalk that warns pedestrians to rush to the safety of the curb.

In a healthy brain, when the orbital frontal cortex warns the brain against heeding reasonable calls to drop a bad habit, it generates anxiety. Anxiety then drives the brain to silence the error warning. Once the error has been corrected, the mistake feeling ends and anxiety disappears. Calm is restored. Thoughts resume their flow from one thing to the next.[25]

When the orbital frontal cortex malfunctions to become overactive, then it causes, in conjunction with other misbehaving brain structures, a condition known as obsessive compulsive disorder (OCD). Those suffering from OCD are tormented by obsessive thoughts and actions that drive them to behave compulsively. People with OCD realize that their compulsive habits are irrational, but still their brain drives them to repeat compulsive behavior.

Jeffrey M. Schwartz, a neuropsychiatrist at the UCLA School of Medicine, has shown that thinking can liberate the brain from the bondage of obsessive compulsive disorder. If people believe that their thoughts have the power to change the brain, and if they exert their wills to break an obsessive habit, then their thoughts alone can alter their brain's physical structure. Daniel Siegel, also of UCLA, agrees. He says that mindful awareness has the power to break habitual thinking.[26]

Thought alters the brain's structure and function

Understanding of the brain's plasticity was initially limited to the discovery that sensory signals from the outside world caused brain cells to wire and rewire themselves. Neuroscience is now finding that sensory signals are not needed to alter the brain's structure. On the contrary, thought alone has the power to change the brain's structure and operation. Signals coming from the brain itself, not from the external environment, can fashion neurons into circuits. As Daniel Siegel, Co-Director of the UCLA Mindful Awareness Research Center, says, "We can actually *focus our minds* in a way that changes the structure and function of the brain throughout our lives."[27]

> "Thought alone has the power to change the brain's structure and operation."

An experiment conducted by Alvaro Pascual-Leone reveals the power of thought to alter the brain. Pascual-Leone invited two groups to learn to play a piano exercise. Neither group of volunteers had ever studied music. Members of one group practiced a five-finger exercise at the piano keyboard. They practiced two hours a day, every day, for five days. Their goal was to play at the metronome's sixty beats per minute without faltering. Brain mapping revealed that at the end of five days, the area of the motor cortex that governed finger movement had expanded. The more the fingers were used, the more space the motor cortex assigned to the fingers.

The other group did not strike keys with their fingers. They sat in front of a piano keyboard, but only imagined that they were hitting the keys. Instead of actually playing five-finger piano exercises, this group played the exercises in their heads for two hours a day for five days. They only imagined how they would move their fingers to generate the notes. Afterwards, brain mapping showed that using imagination to picture raising each finger to play piano exercises expanded the region of the motor cortex that controls the piano-playing fingers. Just as this region had expanded in the brains of those who actually played the piano, so it increased as a result of thought alone. Thinking about the act of playing the piano was by itself sufficient to change neural circuits involved in motor skills. Later on, when those who had only imagined practicing actually used the keyboard, they played as well after two hours as did the group that had practiced the piano for five days. This thought experiment demonstrates that thinking is sufficient to change wiring in the motor region of the brain.[28]

The work of Jeffrey Schwartz also demonstrates that "conscious thoughts and volitions can, and do, play a powerful causal role in . . . influencing the activity of the brain."[29] Believing that thoughts change the brain, Schwartz developed a revolutionary new treatment for OCD that asks patients to think about what their own minds are telling them. People with obsessive compulsive disorder suffer from obsessive thoughts that compel them to perform ritualistic actions. For example, suppose your friend Sam is obsessed with the idea that every time he drives a car, he hits a pedestrian. This obsession causes Sam to imagine, whenever he drives a car, that he hears the thud of hitting someone. This obsession always causes Sam to interrupt his drive and retrace his route. He always retraces his pathway five times to find the imaginary fallen pedestrian. Even as Sam looks for the person he may have run over, the reasoning part of his brain tells him that his car did not hit a pedestrian and that he is wrong to believe that he drove his car into someone.

Schwartz asks his patients to listen to the message coming from the reasoning part of the brain. Reason's message shows them that a broken part of the brain is urging them to act compulsively. They are advised to distinguish between the obsession's false declaration, "Your hands are covered in germs and need to be washed yet again," and reason's true message: "Your hands are clean and do not need to be washed." In making this distinction between the voice of reason and the flawed part of the brain, the patient recognizes that the compulsion is separate from the self. It is an aberration caused by the brain's malfunction.

Patients are then encouraged to resist their obsessive compulsive behavior by replacing it with positive thought and pleasant action. Brain scans show that when Schwartz's patients shift their attention from obeying the compulsion to doing something pleasant, they change the wiring of neurons in their brains, stop the disruptive hyperactivity of the orbital frontal cortex, and become normal. Thinking coupled with doing something pleasant has helped many of Schwartz's patients overcome OCD.[30] Mindful awareness can vanquish automatic habitual thinking.[31]

The power of insubstantial thought to physically sculpt the brain is now being studied in mind-body centers. These centers explore, among other matters, how thought might mitigate stress, depression, and physical pain, and also promote healing. For example, the placebo effect has received considerable attention. Placebos usually help thirty to thirty-five percent of the people who take them. Believing that the placebo is actual medicine, people expect it to work. The belief alone is enough to make the placebo effective.[32]

The power of thought to change the brain's structure is also being explored in studies of Buddhist meditative practices. In *Train Your Mind, Change Your Brain,* Sharon Begley describes research studies involving Buddhists who meditated on compassion. "The meditators' gamma waves were off the charts, and even when the meditators are not meditating, their brains are different from the nonmeditators. . . . " When Buddhists meditated on compassion, brain scans showed "activity in regions responsible for monitoring one's emotions, planning, movements, and positive emotions such as happiness. Regions that keep track of what is 'self' and what is 'other' became quieter, as if, during compassion meditation, the subjects . . . opened their minds and hearts to others."[33]

Research on the meditating Buddhists indicates that "generating a feeling of loving-kindness and compassion has neural correlates in the brains of . . . meditators." When Buddhists meditate on compassion, they produce brain circuits in which compassion is embedded.[34] Their minds create neuronal connections that hold compassion. The research of Martin Seligman, former president of the American Psychological Association, provides further evidence that thinking is by itself sufficient to change the brain's physical state. Seligman showed that when people write down each evening three things that went well that day, eventually they create circuits that hold a grateful attitude. If pessimistic people routinely write down three reasons to be optimistic, in time they will create brain circuits that hold an optimistic outlook.[35]

Thinking changes the brain's physical structure. The lives we lead weave into our neurons the "User's Guide," the Self, that we call "I." Unfortunately, probably most people do not know that their thoughts and experiences shape their brains. Unaware of the power of thought and daily life to alter the brain's structure, people do not worry about examining their mental habits or point of view. Content with their "I," their "User's Guide," they lack the GPS system's ability to acknowledge a mistake and then "recalculate." Those who do not recalculate, who fail to examine the contents of their User's Guide, run on automatic pilot.

Mindfulness

From time to time, probably everyone runs on automatic. A hiker may charge up the steep path intent merely on maintaining his stride and making good time. Hiking on automatic, he misses the color of autumn leaves overhead and the bright sun's reflection on a nearby pond. Often people walk into a meeting thinking, "I've been to meetings like this before; I know what everyone will say, and I know how it will end." Such automatic thoughts lead to automatic conclusions and routine acts.

The automatic, inflexible mind misses daily life. It does not notice new things. It ignores its immediate context, its present circumstances. It minimizes the feelings and thoughts of others. Those coasting on automatic cling to tired beliefs and embrace untested conclusions. As Harvard psychologist Ellen Langer points out, when we run on automatic, instantly we interpret events, hastily we decide what they mean, immediately we judge and reach conclusions about what is going on around us. We defer to authority, continue the same old practices, and fiercely, sometimes violently, protect a long-held idea.[36] We shut the door on understanding ourselves and others. "Living on automatic ... places us at risk of mindlessly reacting to situations without reflecting on various options of response," as Daniel Siegel says. "The result can often be knee-jerk reactions that in turn initiate similar mindless reflexes in others."[37]

Mindfulness, in contrast, allows us to see clearly the world we inhabit. Fully aware, we closely observe our immediate circumstances and are attuned to the thoughts and feelings of others. Observant and interested, we formulate good questions about the present situation, here and now. Asking good questions enables us to gain understanding and insight. Fully aware and keenly attentive, we ask not vague questions such as, "How can we eradicate hunger?" Instead we ask specific questions that address the present moment: "What will it take for our neighborhood to buy and operate a food cart that brings meals to the homeless on Ninth Avenue?"

We need to ask good questions about our immediate context because the questions we ask shape how we live. The human brain is hardwired to extract meaning from the context of daily life. Therefore ask about meaning: "What meaning does this moment hold for me? What understanding might I take away? What meanings will I see? What meanings will I contribute?"

Ask about people: "What does he like to do? What does she worry about?" Consider what it is like to be that person. See with another's eyes; feel with another's heart. Asking good questions leads to life-affirming actions. The Chilean biologist Humberto Maturana observed, "We become the way we live . . .Use context to build yourself. The manner of living leads to the results."[38] The ability to ask good questions depends largely on our ability to pay attention to the moment.

Paying attention

Research in neuroscience suggests that the act of paying attention is essential to the brain's development. Paying keen attention to your son's disappointment triggers mirror neurons that let you share his feeling. Paying attention to the solitary, elderly woman sitting alone on the park bench triggers mirror neurons that let you experience the stranger's loneliness. Paying attention lets us "become the way we live" because it "promotes neural plasticity, the change of neural connections in response to experience."[39] Paying attention to the outside world changes the brain, and paying attention to a thought alters the plastic brain.[40]

Paying attention is a process. The process involves first choosing a target—that is, deciding what specific action, idea, or information merits attention. What will you attend to? Your target may be an insubstantial thought or a tangible object in the outside world. After choosing the target, paying attention involves concentrating on it. When concentration falters, paying attention requires resisting distractions. It requires deflecting irrelevancies and returning attention to the target. William James noted that "voluntarily bringing back a wandering attention, over and over again, is the very root of judgment, character and will."[41] Following this process enables the brain to embed the target in its circuits.

To see how the brain embeds the target in its circuits, imagine that you are paying attention to a chair. Like any object, a chair has many qualities, among them shape and color. One set of neurons is activated when you pay attention to the shape of the chair. A different collection of neurons is affected when you focus on the color of the chair. The neurons that handle color do not talk to the neurons that handle shape. They live in different neighborhoods. This means that if you target shape—if you choose to pay attention only to an object's shape—then you strengthen only the activity of neurons that specialize in shape. Paying attention to shape changes only the specific circuits in the brain dedicated to dealing with shape.[42] Choosing targets intelligently and paying close attention to them changes the plastic, malleable brain. This process helps design the self.

Paying attention means that we are "intentionally aware of what is happening as it is happening, be it sensory processes in the present, or reviewing memories from the past, or plans for the future."[43] Paying attention makes the brain alert, vigilant, and open to what arises. It resists habitual, automatic thinking and develops the capacity to reason.

Recognizing the tremendous power of paying attention, the psychologist and philosopher William James wanted it taught in schools: "An education which would improve this faculty [of attention] would be the education par excellence."[44] Today brain research indicates that children between the ages of three and seven are especially capable of developing the ability to pay attention.[45] At this age, they easily learn to take aim at one target and then stay with it, maintaining attention. Once children gain this skill, it will benefit them for life.

Adults regularly enjoin children to pay attention, usually without explaining how this is done. Ironically, adults are inclined to be inattentive themselves. Rather than pay close attention, they operate on cruise control, depending on information and skills they acquired many years ago. To sharpen their brains, adults need to pay attention as they acquire new knowledge and develop new skills.

Multi-tasking

Dividing attention, known as "multitasking," does not strengthen brain circuits. Today, however, people of all ages, especially adolescents, are multitasking experts. They constantly overlap, cram, and crowd together separate activities. Multitaskers regularly engage at the same time in doing homework, using their "smart phone," watching TV, listening to their ipod, checking e-mail, and text messaging. Research suggests, however, that multitaskers are not really doing many things at the same time. Instead of doing things simultaneously, the brain rapidly shifts attention from one task to the next as it orders these tasks and decides which to handle at any given moment. The practice of shifting attention from one small bit to the next, of dividing attention into small slices, makes it difficult to think deeply and reflect. To live in a state of partial attention, furthermore, always on the alert for a new text message or an exciting bit of information, is to be in a perpetual crisis mode. Inundated with a steady stream of information and trying to balance many things at once, multitaskers experience inordinate stress. Stress causes the brain to produce cortisol, which in the long run impairs cognition. For these reasons, Jordan Grafman, chief of the cognitive neuroscience section of the National Institute of Neurological Disorders and Stroke, predicts that multitaskers will not fare well.[46] The findings of neuroscientists at Stanford University lend support to Grafman's prediction.

Brain research conducted at Stanford University[47] compared multitaskers with students who did not multitask. The performance of multitaskers was not promising. Attuned to search for incoming information, they were easily distracted by the slightest indication that something new might be heading their way. The "ding" that announces, "You've got mail," easily pulled their attention away from the task at hand. They had difficulty keeping things separate in their minds, found it hard to distinguish between what was important and what was trivial, and could not easily tell the relevant from the irrelevant. Students who constantly multitasked apparently damaged their "cognitive control," their control of the thinking process.

Research suggests, then, that multitasking—the mental habit of dividing attention instead of focusing attention on a specific target—discourages reflection, concentration, and clear thinking. The prevalence of multitasking is unfortunate, given how much human kind needs to think deeply and well in this complex twenty-first century.

The ability to reason clearly, assuming it is appropriately balanced with emotion, is humanity's best hope for preserving life and saving Earth. Human beings need to think in a disciplined way to reach sound conclusions that guide them well. In *5 Minds for the Future*, Howard Gardner describes five ways all of us must use our brains if society is to thrive in the future. He points out the importance of being disciplined enough to master a subject, of being skilled at synthesizing information from disparate sources, of being creative, respectful, and ethical.[48] My modest focus is on thinking about thinking, which I call "critical thinking." Critical thinking helps us gain the fullest understanding possible, and it helps us moderate the potentially overpowering influence of emotion.[49]

Critical Thinking

The term "critical" thinker means a meticulous thinker who wants to completely understand any issue or situation. Twenty-first century Americans, however, seem unwilling to "respect different views, weigh them, vote for the ones that make the most sense, and abide by majority rule while respecting minority rights." Ironically, in America, the home of democracy, political and social issues seem increasingly to be decided by passion, bribes, and lies, not reason.[50] Many people do think scrupulously and critically, of course, about education, the economy, and social policies. Many are receptive, open-minded, and honest in their pursuit of knowledge. Such critical thinkers regard thinking as a rigorous activity that leads to understanding. They systematically examine the reasoning behind arguments, claims, opinions, and convictions. They scrutinize their own ideas and those of others to see if these ideas are worth keeping. Critical thinkers focus on hard facts, scrutinize evidence to see if it is reliable, notice relationships among data, dissect claims, synthesize information, and try to anticipate the consequences of any conclusions they reach. Critical thinkers ask thoughtful questions, such as:

1. What is the issue, problem or project under discussion?

2. What is your own point of view? Are you biased? Set aside your biases. Is the other person biased? Notice her biases.

3. What reasons support a position? Do they follow from one another logically?

4. Do hard facts support the reasoning?

5. What evidence is available to underpin the reasons given? Why do you think the evidence is reliable?

6. Does the language hold meaning? Does it make sense?

7. What conclusions are offered? Do they follow logically from the reasons?

8. What side-effects might arise if a conclusion is accepted? What unanticipated consequences might arise?

9. Given the side-effects, does the conclusion merit endorsement or adoption?

Today inquiry tends to be driven by unexamined opinions and convictions, not by skilled and honest reason used to achieve insight, truth, and wisdom. It is essential that parents and educators recognize a responsibility to help children become critical thinkers who value and search for understanding and truth, however elusive these might be.

Thinking well and being mindful of others—seeing others non-judgmentally in the fullness of their unique being—leads to enlightened morality. Enlightened morality approaches every experience with the qualities of mindfulness that Daniel Siegel calls COAL, "curiosity, openness, acceptance, and love."[51] Enlightened morality assigns equal value to all people. It sees all people as equally entitled to health, happiness, security, and opportunities to develop their full promise. Enlightened morality treats others as one wishes to be treated; it is love.

Chapter 5: Endnotes

1. Thomas Lewis, Fari Amini, Richard Lannon, *A General Theory of Love* (New York: Vintage, 2000), pp. 124-144. The brain frames H in the sense that it extracts "H-ness" from any version of that letter. It has an ingrained prototype of H. "Prototype extraction—the distillation of pure, intoxicating principles from the muddle of diverse experiences—is the natural inescapable outcome of neural memory." p. 136.

2. Lewis, Amini, Lannon, p. 141. Daniel Levitin points out in *This is Your Brain on Music* (New York: Plume, 2006), pp. 232-235 that by the age of eighteen our musical tastes are set—our cognitive schema is wired. The schema is "the system into which we place" our understanding of a piece of music. It "frames our understanding.". In the same way, ideas are wired into the brain and frame our understanding of new information.

3. Steven Pinker, "The Moral Instinct," *The New York Times Magazine,* (January 13, 2009) <http://www.nytimes.com/2008/01/13/magazine/13Psychology-t.hjtml>.

4. Paul Bloom, "The Moral Life of Babies," *The New York Times* (3 May 2010), pp. 2, 3-5. <http://www.nytimes.com/2010/05/09/magazine/09babies>.

5. See Gazzaniga, *Human* (New York: HarperCollins, 2008) p. 130; Steven Pinker, "The Moral Instinct," *The New York Times*, pp. 7-8, for remarks on Hauser's five universal "moral modules . . . reciprocity, suffering, hierarchy, . . . coalitions, and purity."

6. Jeffrey Kluger, "What Makes Us Moral," *Your Brain: A User's Guide*, ed. Jeffrey Kluger (New York: Time, Inc., 2009), p. 84: "The deepest foundation on which morality is built is the phenomenon of empathy . . . ."

7. Pinker, "The Moral Instinct," *The New York Times*, p. 6.

8. On empathy in Rhesus monkeys see Daniel Goleman, *Social Intelligence* (New York: Bantam Books, 2006), pp. 55-56. Jeffrey Kluger discusses in "What Makes Us Moral?" *Your Brain* p. 86, the gorilla Binta Jua's empathetic rescue in 1996 of a three-year old boy. Kluger also discusses Russian primatologist Nadia Kohts' study of empathy in young chimpanzees.

9. Gazzaniga, *Human,* p. 133; Pinker, "The Moral Instinct," *The New York Times,* p. 8.

10. Michael Shermer, "Don't Be Evil: Enron, Google and the Evolutionary Psychology of Corporate Environment, *Scientific American Mind* (February/March, 2008), pp. 59-65.

11. Gazzaniga, *Human,* pp. 136-137.

12. Interestingly, recent work in physics and biology qualifies the idea that humankind is innately hierarchical. Astrophysics in particular suggests that all things, living and non-living, human and non-human, are interdependent members of the universe, itself a system of subsystems. The interdependence permeating the universe unites all things into a web of relationships in which each part is equal in value to the rest and each is essential to produce a whole that exceeds the sum of its parts. An innate disposition to empathy, not an innate disposition to defer to those who may legitimately claim authority, is implicit in interdependence.

13. Gazzaniga, *Human,* p. 137.

14. Jeffrey Kluger, "What Makes Us Moral" *Time* (December 3, 2007), pp. 54-60. See also for a related study of this topic: Kluger, "What Makes Us Moral?" *Your Brain: A User's Guide,*" pp 84-88.

15. John B. Cobb, Jr. "Capital," a paper written for a conference in Suzhou, China (January 2009), pp. 4-13. Cobb provides a careful description of the power of privately owned commercial banks and of the Federal Reserve Bank in particular, owned and run by commercial banks.

16. Gazzaniga, *Human*, pp. 143-144 cites Robert Wright's *The Moral Animal*. Wright notes that the human brain, like any lawyer, wants to win. "Given any set of interests to defend, it [the brain]. . . sets about convincing the world of their moral and logical worth regardless of whether they in fact have any of either. . ."

17. See Carter, *Mapping the Mind*, p. 108: "An individual's view is formed both by their genes and by how their brain has been moulded by experience."

18. Prof. Ann Greybiel made this observation in a lecture delivered as part of the OHSU Brain Awareness Lecture Series, Portland, Oregon, 23 Oct. 2002.

19. Rita Carter, Susan Aldridge, Martyn Page, Steve Parker, *The Human Brain Book* (New York: D. K. Publishing, 2009), p. 226.

20. Nikolas Westerhoff, "Set in Our Ways," *Scientific American Mind* (Dec/Jan. 2009), pp. 44-49. Westerhoff cites Gerhard Roth of the University of Bremen, author of *Personality, Decision, and Behavior* (2007).

21. Jeffrey M. Schwartz and Sharon Begley, *The Mind and the Brain* (New York: Regan Books, 2002), pp. 61-73, 69, fig. 2: TAN nerve cells in the basal ganglia integrate reason and emotion; David Rock and Jeffrey Schwartz, "The Neuroscience of Leadership," *Strategy + Business* (Summer, 2006) issue 43, p. 4.

22. Ken Currier, "Why are Bad Habits so Hard to Break?" *Stuff Your Brain Likes* (27 May 2008) http://www.stuffyourbrainlikes.com; Maia Szalavitz, "Kindness 101," *Time* (May 24, 2010), p. 46. On the basal ganglia, see Rita Carter, *Mapping the Mind*, pp. 56-60; David Rock and Jeffrey Schwartz, "The Neuroscience of Leadership," pp. 2-10; Elkhonen Goldberg, *The Executive Brain: Frontal Lobes and the Civilized Mind* (Oxford: Oxford University Press, 2001), p. 180. Jeffrey M. Schwartz and Sharon Begley, *The Mind and the Brain*, pp. 68-71. The part of the basal ganglia called the caudate nucleus exchanges signals with two important areas in the prefrontal cortex: the anterior cingulate gyrus and the orbital frontal cortex. It is "at the confluence of messages bearing cognitive content . . . where inputs arrive from the rational prefrontal cortex and message . . . with emotion. . . from the limbic system. . . .TAN cells in the basal ganglia integrate information from the limbic system and the prefrontal cortex." pp. 68-69.

23. Alvaro Pascual-Leone, cited in Norman Doidge, *The Brain that Changes Itself* (New York: Viking, 2007), pp. 209-211.

24. Nickolas Westerhoff, pp. 44-49.

25. Schwartz and Begley, *The Mind and the Brain*, pp. 63-70.

26. The orbital frontal circuit consisting of the orbital frontal cortex, anterior cingulate gyrus and caudate nucleus enforces habits. The anterior cingulate cortex focuses attention and regulates emotional arousal (Siegel, 114). These habits can be broken by "the exertion of willful effort." Schwartz and Begley, *The Mind and the Brain*, p. 94.

27. Daniel Siegel. *The Mindful Brain*," (New York: W.Norton & Co., 2007), p. 96. See also Sharon Begley, "How the Brain Rewires Itself," *Time*, (January 29, 2007), pp. 68-74.

28. Sharon Begley, *Train Your Mind, Change Your Brain* (New York: Ballantine Books, 2007), pp. 151-152; Sharon Begley, "How the Brain Rewires Itself," pp. 68-74. Norman Doidge, *The Brain that Changes itself* (New York: Viking, 2007), pp.201-202.

29. Schwartz, M.D. and Begley, *The Mind and the Brain*, pp. 16-17.

30. Sharon Begley, *Train Your Mind, Change Your Brain* (New York: Ballantine Books, 2007), pp. 137-141; Schwartz and Begley, pp. 18-50; Mario Beauregard and Denyse O'Leary, *The Spiritual Brain* (New York: Harper One, 2007), pp. 126-131.

31. Daniel J. Siegel, *The Mindful Brain* (New York: W.W. Norton & Company, 2007), p. 115.

32. Mario Beauregard and Denyse O'Leary, *The Spiritual Brain* (New York: Harper One, 2007), pp. 141-150; Begley, *Train Your Mind, Change Your Brain,* pp. 141-150; Doidge, *The Brain that Changes Itself* pp. 201-202.

33. Begley, *Train Your Mind, Change Your Brain*, pp. 235.

34. Begley, *Train Your Mind, Change Your Brain*, p. 237.

35. Seligman cited in David Rock and Jeffrey Schwartz, p. 9.

36. Ellen J. Langer, *The Power of Mindful Learning* (Cambridge: Perseus Books, 1997), pp. 16-18,100, 103-105: "What is out there is shaped by how we view it." See also C. Otto Scharmer. *Theory U* (San Francisco: Berrett-Koehler, 2009), pp. 119-121; *Theory U's* Foreword by management theorist Peter Senge, p.xiii.

37. Daniel J. Siegel, *The Mindful Brain* (New York: W. W. Norton & Company, 2007), p. 14.

38. Humberto Maturana and Pille Bunnell. "Biosphere, Homosphere, and Robosphere: What Has That to do with Business?" Paper based on a presentation made by Humberto Maturana at the Society for Organizational Learning Member's Meeting, Amherst, MA, June, 1998, edited by Pille Bunnell. **http://www.sol-ne.org/res/wp/maturana.** Downloaded January 27, 1999. See also, Humberto Maturana and Pille Bunnell, "The Biology of Business: Love Expands Intelligence," *Reflections,* volume 1, number 2.

39. Siegel, p. 25.

40. Siegel, pp. 110-111. "There is not just one form of attention. . . . There are three generally agreed upon aspects: . . .executive, orienting, and alerting." Attention networks in the cortical and subcortical networks mediate these aspects of attention.

41. William James, *The Principles of Psychology,* cited in Siegel, p. 266.

42. Begley, *Train Your Mind, Change Your Brain*, p. 157.

43. Siegel, p. 267.

44. William James, *Principles of Psychology* (1890), cited in Siegel, p. 266.

45. Siegel, p. 115; See also p. 112, "attention is a trainable skill" p. 114: "attention can decouple automatic habitual thinking."

46. Claudia Wallis. "Gen M: The Multitasking Generation," *Time* (March 27, 2006), pp. 48-58; Gary Small and Gigi Vorgan, "Meet Your Brain," *Scientific American Mind* (July/August 2008), pp. 42-49.

47. For an account of the Stanford experiment see, Matt Richtel, "Hooked on Gadgets, and Paying a Mental Price," *The New York Times* (June 7, 2010) http://www.nytimes. com/2010/06/07, downloaded June 10, 2010. *Computer World* www.computerworld.com. (September 1, 2009) describes research by Stanford professors Clifford Nass, Eyal Ophir, and Anthony Wagner.

48. Howard Gardner, *5 Minds for the Future* (Boston: Harvard Business Press, 2008), pp. xiii-xv.

49. On multitasking see, for example, Christine Rosen. "The Myth of Multitasking," in the *New Atlantis: A Journal of Technology & Society.* (Spring, 2008), No. 20, pp. 105-110. <www. thenewatlantis.com>

50. Donella Meadows, "Voice of a Global Citizen," <www.sustainabilityinstitute.org/DHM archive/index> 5 J08.

51. Siegel, p. 15.

CHAPTER 6

Shaping a Brain-Friendly
Learning Environment

"The degree to which we are all involved in the control
of the earth's life is just beginning to dawn on most of us,
and it means another revolution for human thought."

Lewis Thomas. *Natural Man, The Lives of a Cell.* 1974.

"I believe . . . In singing, especially when
singing is not necessarily prescribed."

Mary Oliver. *Evidence.*

"Give about two [hours] every day to exercise; for health must not
be sacrificed to learning. A Strong body makes the mind strong."

Thomas Jefferson. *Letter to Peter Carr.* 19 August 1785.

KNOWING ABOUT THE BRAIN'S STRUCTURE AND OPERATION
naturally raises a very important question: What kind of environment is best for the human brain? During the past thirty years,
neuroscientists have proved that the brain is malleable, not rigid
and inert. They have shown that environment, signaling the brain
by way of the five senses, causes brain cells to connect and re-con-
nect. They have also discovered, remarkably, that thought alone
strengthens existing connections—synapses—and makes new

ones. Every day, both thoughts and environment sculpt the brain. The monumentally important discovery that thinking and experiences shape the brain compels us to think carefully about the kind of environment that we and our children inhabit.

Because environment and thought change the brain's physical structure, we benefit from brain-friendly homes, schools, workplaces and communities. Brain friendly conditions shape brain circuits that hold knowledge, skills, ideas, and attitudes that will secure a safe and gracious future for the individual, benefit the community, and protect Earth. This chapter considers some characteristics of a brain-friendly environment, such as the study of music, physical exercise, reasoning well, governing emotions, paying attention, cultivating mindfulness, and developing positive relationships. It also discusses the effects on society of digital technology. Are digital inventions changing the brain's structure for better or worse? Does violent entertainment produce violent brains?

Music: the Brain's Friend

Music deserves a prominent place in a brain-friendly environment. Until the 1980s, neuroscience had not looked carefully at the effects of music on the brain. Today, thanks to new technology, scientists have hard evidence that music affects virtually every region of the brain and every brain function.[1] Neuroscience reveals that music is far from being an incidental, inconsequential activity. It grows and strengthens the brain.

Human beings are born to make and appreciate music. Just as humans have an innate ability to acquire language, so they have an innate capacity to learn music. Children understand music as naturally and easily as they master their native language. During the first few years of life, the child's brain readily wires for music of any kind. For instance, children in the United States and Europe hear western music and therefore their brains form neural circuits that hold western sounds. For that reason, five-year olds can tell if a song or melody from their culture breaks a structural rule.

Music has such a powerful impact on the young brain that just listening to music is by itself sufficient to strengthen existing neural circuits and add new ones. Hearing a new song, for instance, causes the brain to respond by wiring a neural pathway. When it wires this new pathway, the brain strengthens its auditory cortex and thus makes hearing more acute.[2] Listening to music also improves the capacity of the planum temporale, the brain's sound-signal processor, to detect the rise and fall of pitch. In addition to sharpening an awareness of pitch, hearing songs sharpens timbre and rhythm. Listening to music also strengthens a child's ability to remember music.

Although listening to music benefits the brain in many ways, the benefits of making music, of playing an instrument, are greater still. MRIs of the brains of musicians show the impact on the brain of playing an instrument. In the brains of musicians, the area in the auditory cortex that is wired expressly to process music is twenty-five percent larger than in the brains of non-musicians. Musicians are therefore able to hear nuances in music that elude most of us. In a trumpeter's brain, for example, more space is dedicated to "brassy" sounds than is found in the brains of non-trumpeters.[3]

Playing an instrument engages not only the auditory cortex, but also many other brain regions. A specific part of the motor cortex, for example, controls movement of fingers on the violinist's left hand. This area grows larger—the density and power of neurons in this part of the motor cortex increases—the more the violinist practices. Young people learning to play also develop spatial awareness, good memories, and the ability to coordinate complex movements.

To control coordination and balance, the cerebellum works with the motor cortex. In addition, the cerebellum, "the little brain," cooperates with the basal ganglia, the brain's habit center, to store the technical skills that musicians acquire through practice. Patterns of activity basic to playing an instrument thus become stored as automatic memory.

The person who begins playing an instrument before the age of seven, furthermore, has an unusually large corpus callosum, the fiber that connects the two cerebral hemispheres and makes it possible for them to communicate. Because the musician's corpus callosum is enlarged, it is able to carry more information between the hemispheres than would normally be the case. This heightened communication helps unify, in other words, the two sides of the brain.

Playing an instrument while reading music enlists the help, among other areas, of the part of the cortex known as the parietal lobe. Among its many functions, the parietal lobe handles spatial awareness. Neural circuits in the parietal lobe help the musician recognize and interpret spatial relationships among notes on a musical staff. The frontal lobe, the thinking part of the brain, is engaged constantly as a musician reads music and practices. Learning to play a musical instrument cultivates and increases the frontal lobe's ability to pay attention, analyze symbols, use logic, solve problems, and make comparisons.[4]

Studying music does more than build brain regions essential to intellectual and physical prowess. It also generates qualities that build character. To become a musician requires, for example, patience, determination, the ability to learn from mistakes, persistence, and self-confidence. In addition to wiring the brain with these and other attributes, the study of music contributes to a sociable brain. Although learning an instrument typically involves a great deal of solitary work, making and listening to music are typically highly social activities. When musicians play together, it is as though their minds communicate telepathically. Furthermore, music's universal language is emotion. When many people listen to the same song, they share identical emotions. These shared emotions unite them. Music also causes people to have a sense of belonging as they dance and sing together, moving their muscles in the same way.[5]

Music deserves to be studied for its own sake, as well as because it engages virtually every region of the brain, builds character, and unites people. Music sustains and inspires human beings. It soothes, energizes, calms, and enlightens us. Music ignites the soul. Every child deserves to learn music.

The preschooler's brain-friendly world

Neuroscience makes it clear—and teaching successes in Europe confirm– that very young children are ready for exposure to music and a second language. Experience and research show that children in elementary school more easily learn music and the syntax of a second language than do high school students. In fact, by late adolescence, the window of opportunity for easily learning music and syntax closes.

Although very young children naturally respond when they hear languages and music, it is not clear that their brains are ready for challenging academic training. The brains of three and four-year olds may not benefit from being asked, as they are in many preschools, to memorize answers to arithmetic problems or spell words on flash cards. Because children's flexible, plastic brains make neural connections easily, children may accomplish difficult academic tasks. However, the question remains: Is there a cost involved?

If the young brain has not yet developed the neural networks suitable to deal naturally with an academic assignment, the child's brain might rely on inappropriate neural systems to work out the answer to an arithmetic problem. Lessons that make premature demands on the developing brain and thus force it to use inappropriate neural systems might eventually interfere with the brain's natural development.

If demanding academic material is presented too early in life, it might cause children not only intellectual, but also emotional problems. Asked too soon to add, subtract, or read, very young children might feel insecure, confused, and uncertain of their own ability to learn. They might experience damaging stress. If pre-schoolers are not able to attach meaning to premature lessons, fur-thermore, they cannot build on them.

For these reasons, it may be unwise to risk making *premature* academic demands on young brains. Until more research is done on how early academic training affects brain development, it might be wise to substitute for an academic preschool a brain-friendly environment that nurtures the whole child. It has been shown that children benefit when they receive individual attention, talk often with one adult, and are encouraged to do such things as practice self-control, listen, learn songs, explain why they think something is true, think about what something means, use imagination, exer-cise, pay attention, cooperate with others, and socialize. Such expe-riences sculpt circuits that will endure for a lifetime and affect the kind of adult a preschooler becomes.[6]

Physical activity strengthens the brain

Research indicates that for adults and children alike, a brain-friendly environment includes frequent and regular physical exercise. Common sense has always told us that exercise is good for the body. Thanks to neuroscience, we now know that exercise is also good for the brains of young and old alike. Aerobic exercise—running, walk-ing briskly, cycling, jumping, swimming, playing basketball or soc-cer (but without head-butting the ball)—causes the growth of new blood vessels and increases blood flow to the brain, thus increasing the brain's supply of oxygen and nutrition. Research shows that aerobic exercise also causes new brain cells to grow in the part of the hippocampus known as the dentate gyrus, an area essential to memory, and in the olfactory region.

"Music and physical activity grow and strengthen the brain."

Dr. Fred Gage and his colleagues at the Laboratory of Genetics at the Salk Institute in San Diego showed in the 1990s that neurogenesis—the growth of new brain cells—does occur and that exercise stimulates this growth. A variety of subsequent experiments conducted by scientists at the Salk Institute, the Feinberg School of Medicine in Chicago, Columbia University, and Harvard Medical School confirm the discovery that exercise produces new brain cells. In fact, engaging in aerobic exercise from thirty minutes to one hour on four consecutive days each week stimulates the birth of new brain cells, increases blood volume, sharpens memory and mental acuity, and helps ensure that neuronal stem cells stay lively.[7] Aerobic exercise, according to a persuasive Swedish study published in 2009, seems to stimulate the brain and raise IQ. The Swedish study found that the eighteen-year olds who engaged vigorously in aerobic exercise attained higher IQs than did those eighteen-year olds who went without exercise.[8]

Physical activity is good for any brain, regardless of age. Exercise helps preschoolers understand their own capacities and interpret their surroundings.[9] In nine and ten year olds, studies show, exercise increases the size of distinct brain regions and in so doing may enhance cognition.[10] Specifically, when nine- and ten-year olds exercise, the size of their basal ganglia increases. This increase is significant because the basal ganglia, which affects motor control and holds habits, influences the coordination not only of actions, but also of thoughts. Furthermore, when youth exercise, the hippocampus, the gateway to the long-term memory, grows in size and becomes more active. The basal ganglia and hippocampus collaborate to aid subtle thinking. Scientists have found that at any age taking a daily walk benefits the brain by increasing connections among brain circuits.

Researchers from the Karolinska Institute in Stockholm spent thirty-five years studying the effects of exercise on 1,500 people. They learned that people who exercised were far less subject to dementia than were sedentary people. Scientists in Hawaii reached a similar conclusion. Their study of 2,000 elderly men living in Hawaii found that vigorous exercise keeps the brain alert and sharp.[11] Because exercise strengthens memory, improves cognition, causes the growth of new cells, and forestalls dementia, exercise should be an integral part of daily life from youth to old age.

Sleep

Just as aerobic exercise is essential for the brain's health, so is sleep. Sleep is as necessary to the healthy brain as nourishment and oxygen. While we sleep, the brain keeps working. During sleep, the brain works hard to make proteins, store essential chemicals, and assure supplies of energy and oxygen. Constantly firing, neurons in the sleeping brain also make connections that affect learning, insight, memory, and motor skills. If you are learning to type or play tennis, for example, after practicing that skill, make certain to get a good night's sleep. During sleep, your brain will strengthen the new physical skill. Asleep, the brain also reviews, compares, contrasts, and analyzes newly acquired information. When it sees meaning in new information, it tends to store it in the long-term memory. Sometimes the sleeping brain solves perplexing problems that clouded the day. It is not unusual to awaken to discover that during sleep, we generated a new idea or insight. While we sleep, the brain performs many necessary and remarkable functions.

Therefore a brain-friendly environment sees to it that people have the time and opportunity to get a good night's sleep.[12]

Reason and emotion connected

Neuroscientists have made two fascinating discoveries that affect how we regard thought and emotion. They discovered that more signals travel from the brain's emotional center to the reasoning area than move in the opposite direction. Because signaling is weighted in favor of emotion, emotion often has the power to overwhelm rational thought. Neuroscientists also discovered that thought alone is by itself sufficient to cause brain cells to forge connections. Taken together, these astonishing discoveries make it urgent that young people be taught to think well. Thinking well involves systematic reasoning that balances reason with emotion and leads to logical, informed conclusions. Thinking well is also an act of mindfulness. Mindfulness requires being open to whatever is happening at any moment; it means paying full and explicit attention to the moment.

A brain-friendly environment encourages people to manage their emotions and trains them to think about the thinking process itself. It helps them cultivate awareness and escape running on automatic pilot.

Building positive relationships

One of the most remarkable features of the brain is its sociable nature. Social to the core, the human brain flourishes when other brains like, admire, respect, and appreciate it—when it belongs. Human beings are joyful when they belong and suffer great social pain when they are spurned. It is imperative, therefore, that we create a brain-friendly community that nurtures accepting, respectful, and kind relationships. Simple acts of consideration and kindness, such as listening attentively and replying courteously, create an environment that helps people relate to others and feel they belong.

In shaping a welcoming and safe environment, it is helpful to remember that because the human brain possesses mirror neurons, human beings "watch and wire." Children do this with great alacrity. Mirror neurons let children easily perform in their own brains the actions and attitudes they observe. When children watch a teacher show patience and tolerance to a classmate, the child's mirror neurons readily imitate the patience and tolerance evident in the teacher's behavior. Hearing a teacher speak in a sarcastic and belittling voice activates the child's mirror neurons to replicate that belittling sarcasm. When adults are kind, fully present to others, accept and include everyone, and provide secure and safe surroundings, children watch, wire, and become like these adults.

A brain-friendly environment not only provides mirror neurons with behavior worth emulating, but also it builds relationships. It encourages children, for instance, to interact with their peers in person, face-to-face. For example, a friend's eleven-year old son, fictitiously named Mark, came home from school and boasted happily that as a practical joke he had tampered with his pal Jeff's smart phone. Mark's parents anticipated that the joke might upset Mark's friend. They told Mark to contact Jeff immediately to explain what he had done.

Mark said, "O.K., I'll text him."

His parents said, "No, please go to Jeff's house. You need to talk to him in person."

The parents were wise, brain research indicates, to ask Mark to face Jeff in person. In a one-on-one meeting, facial expressions, eye contact, gestures, movements, and tone of voice send a variety of sensory signals that enrich and clarify mutual understanding. A person-to-person encounter, furthermore, calls for civility and tact. Speaking face-to-face discourages behaving in a cavalier, flippant, or indifferent way. It discourages treating someone as an object or terminating a conversation abruptly. When they talked in person, Mark and Jeff were responsive to one another and fully present. Furthermore, the genial atmosphere of the place where they talked—Jeff's kitchen—positively influenced their conversation. Mark returned home pleased that Jeff had appreciated his practical joke and confident that he and Jeff remained excellent friends.

A brain-friendly environment values life-enhancing relationships. Modern physics and biology tell us that we are actually interdependent, not independent, members of one web of life. Today neuroscience tells us that mirror neurons form circuits that hold both what we observe, and what we do. When we observe and engage in kind, caring relationships, the brain thrives.

Digital technology and relationships

In 1999, the National Institute of Mental Health (NIMH) discredited the long-held position of neuroscience that the teenage brain had slight plasticity compared with the plasticity of a young child's brain. NIMH discovered that the adolescent brain actually possesses enormous plasticity. This finding means that a teenager's behavior can dramatically change the architecture of his or her brain.

The plasticity of the adolescent brain is a mixed blessing. It enables the teenager's brain to wire and rewire easily in response to an enriched environment that strengthens it. However, it also enables the adolescent brain just as easily to form circuits in response to an impoverished environment that diminishes it. When teenagers observe adults exerting self-discipline to achieve goals, their own brains generate circuits that hold self-discipline. When teenagers spend quality time in the company of adults who appreciate and respect them, their brains wire feelings of security and confidence. When adolescents are with adults who treat others with kindness, compassion, and courtesy, their mirror neurons wire for kindness, respect and empathy.[13]

Increasingly, however, teenagers and adults are becoming distanced from one another. One reason for this distance is that adolescents spend about forty percent of their time using computers, e-mail, Facebook, cell phones, text messaging, twittering, playing video games, and watching movies and television. The time they devote to these devices reduces, of course, the time they might spend with adults.

Teenagers are not alone, as it happens, in choosing to concentrate on electronic devices rather than on family and friends. Five years of research by the MIT Initiative on Technology and Self shows that parents are increasingly choosing to immerse themselves in a digital world at the expense of their children. Many parents ignore their children to attend to cell phones, instant messaging, and email. Deprived of their parents' attention, children feel hurt and lonely.[14]

Although some parent's routinely neglect their children in the interests of using electronic devices like cell phones and computers, other parents inadvertently cut themselves off from their children by remaining ignorant of these electronic devices that fascinate the young. Uninterested in Facebook or Twitter, indifferent to the smart phone, these parents condemn themselves to pacing on the sidelines of their children's lives. If adults will not speak the electronic language of the twenty-first century, how can they interact with young people?

Is digital technology brain-friendly?

Digital technology so powerfully influences every facet of contemporary life that neuroscientists are concerned about its impact on the brain. To alter the brain is to alter the species. Presumably everyone, then, should pay attention to the neural sculpting of the human brain that results from immersion in digital technology.

From the age of eight to eighteen, young people in the United States typically spend about eight hours a day using some kind of electronic device. Consequently, their brains are wired differently from the brains of adults. As a result of deep immersion in electronic technology, teenagers' brains are wired, for instance, to respond quickly to flashes of light and color, instantly to interpret visual stimuli, and rapidly to gather and sort through huge quantities of information on the internet. Do electronic devices also wire brains to concentrate, postpone gratification, consider long-term consequences, empathize, think critically, and interpret gestures and facial expressions? Are they brain- friendly? The next section considers the effects on the human brain of television, movies, and video games. We begin by asking if video games belong in a brain-friendly environment.[15]

Video games: positive and negative features

Research shows that video games affect players in both positive and negative ways. The positive effects of playing video games are wide-ranging and impressive. When my son was four years old, for instance, his physical therapist supervised him in hours of video gaming that strengthened his fine motor control, hand-eye coordination, perception of spatial relationships, and reflexes. Video games have also been found to improve the brain's visual processing pathway. Daphne Bavelier, a professor of brain and cognitive sciences, found that playing fast-paced video games for fifty hours over a period of nine weeks helped patients better distinguish between shades of gray.[16]

In addition to helping people see contrasts, develop physical reflexes, sharpen spatial orientation, and improve hand-eye coordination, video games strengthen mental abilities. Video games are elaborate puzzles containing secret rules and hidden strategies. The player's task is to figure out these rules and strategies. To this end, the player is a problem solver. He solves problems by using trial and error and formulating a hypothesis. The player instinctively uses, in other words, the scientific method. Not only intellectual capacities, but also personality traits can be positively shaped by playing video games. To succeed, video gamers must be determined to recover from failure, persevere, and exercise self-discipline.[17]

It may be, however, that playing video games wires brains in undesirable ways. Critics of video games blame them, among other things, for being devoid of content and meaning. Players focus exclusively on achieving the goal. They concentrate on the means that will lead to the desired end. The single goal of the video gamer is to accomplish the task at hand, whether that objective is to win the battle or rescue the princess from a tower. The player's focus is exclusively on getting the job done. If the purpose of the game is to win the battle, the player's thrill comes from doing so. The game does not ask the player to wonder, "Why is this battle happening? Is it just?" The meaning of the battle is irrelevant. If the goal is to rescue the princess from the tower, the player's thrill comes from saving her. The game does not ask the player to consider why the princess is locked in the tower in the first place. Maybe she is a serial killer and her family keeps her in the tower to protect society. It does not matter. The story is irrelevant in video games. Meaning and content have no place. All that matters is reaching the goal by any means possible.

Because video games focus only on steps leading to success and not on meaningful content, they do not offer the prefrontal cortex substantive information that provides a foundation for informed thought. The more time people spend playing video games, the less time they dedicate to acquiring the skills and knowledge essential to navigate in this complex world.

The pleasure that gamers derive from concentrating on video games, furthermore, disposes their brains to be content with rewards produced by empty accomplishments. When Pac Man devours a ball or evades a ghost, the player's reward circuit is activated. The activated reward circuit causes the release of dopamine, which generates a feeling of pleasure. Because the reward circuit's pleasurable feeling is so satisfying, people seek to replicate it. Wanting to repeat the pleasure, the gamer gets hooked on playing the game. Playing a video game to trigger the brain's release of dopamine makes trivial use of the brain's reward system. The brain would be better served, of course, were its reward system triggered by real-world activities such as doing well on an examination, gaining a skill, or enjoying the company of good friends.

Another problem with video games is that the programmer makes the rules, rules that are necessarily inviolate. Because video games require adherence to their rules, they inculcate compliance rather than originality and creativity. Only if players conform to the game's rules and requirements will they succeed. Players cannot challenge a game. They must "always . . . accept the system and work to succeed within it."[18] Deferring to the rules, following orders, and patiently climbing the ladder to the next level are perquisites for gaming success. Young people looking at an electronic screen are permitted only to ask questions decreed by the game itself. They have no opportunity to ask imaginative questions.

Violent video games wire the brain

Despite their drawbacks, some video games serve a constructive purpose that aids learning. Some games do have a place in a brain-friendly environment. Violent video games, however, according to brain research, have no place in a brain-friendly environment. Neuroscience shows that the virtual violence generated to entertain youth generates violent minds.

Playing violent video games requires participating in violent acts. Players decide to smash a man in the head or shoot a woman. Those who spend hours in front of a screen stalking, beating, and stabbing realistic images of human beings are building neuronal circuits in their malleable brains that embed violent acts and condone violent behavior. The brain's neurons do not distinguish between pretend violence and real violence. Neurons do not say, "This action is pretend, so we will not connect to form a circuit." If a player shoots a virtual man using a virtual gun, his brain acts as if he had shot a real person using a real gun. His brain builds real circuits that dispose him to act violently in the real world.

> "The brain's neurons do not distinguish between pretend violence and real violence."

Spending hours violently subduing virtual human beings causes players, furthermore, to discount the value of an individual life. Gaming wires their brains to dismiss real people as expendable objects. When a video game attaches success to violent action, as does "Grand Theft Auto," the effect on the player's brain is especially insidious. Violence that results often in success forges circuits that become embedded with the conviction that harming someone is a defensible career move, or that injuring another is permissible in the service of a righteous end. Violence, players learn, is a legitimate means to a desired end.[19]

It is also important to realize that when a video gamer simulates murder and replicates physical assault hour after hour, the player impairs the brain's ability to limit aggressiveness. Repeated immersion in violent video games reduces the power of the anterior cingulate cortex to inhibit aggressive behavior, monitor conduct, and exercise self-control.

Violence on television and in movies

Video games are not the only entertainment, of course, that wires the malleable human brain to regard violence as ordinary and acceptable. By the time the typical young person in the U.S. reaches the age of eighteen, he or she will have watched on television or in movies more than 200,000 acts of violence, including more than 16,000 murders. Neuroscience has discovered that depictions of violence in movies and on television alter the brain's physical structure in ways that increase the probability that children will eventually behave violently.[20]

According to neuroscientist Marco Iacoboni, a pioneer in the study of mirror neurons, decisive evidence proves that watching violence portrayed in movies and on television wires mirror neurons to imitate violence.[21] Moreover, according to Iacoboni's laboratory and longitudinal studies, these "mirror neurons in our brains produce *automatic* imitative influences . . . *that limit our autonomy.*"[22] In other words, our brain's mirror neurons encode in circuits the specific *virtual* violent actions that we observe in a movie. These circuits then become a kind of template for future use. This template makes it easy for the movie-goer, weeks, months, or years later, to enact in real life the violent behavior observed long ago on a screen. It is a disquieting fact that when young people passively watch violence on television and in movies, they are actually changing their brain's physical structure to facilitate violent acts.

Not surprisingly, the entertainment industry resists criticism of the violence that it finds so profitable. Predictably, adolescents also resist objections to violent entertainment. Quick to dismiss warnings that violent video games and violence on the screen will wire their brains for future violent behavior, typically young people say, "I know that what I'm watching isn't real. Pretend violence doesn't fool me into approving of real-life violence. Besides, although I have played violent games hundreds of times and have viewed countless violent movies and television programs, I'm still a good person. I would never hurt anybody." What people do not realize is that interactive video games and countless scenes of violence have created circuits in their brains that predispose them to act violently. The right catalytic agent might trigger these circuits to initiate violent behavior.

Screen time for children: brain friendly?

Violence is not the only reason to be wary of the electronic screens that entertain us. Using television to baby-sit infants and toddlers adversely affects the growing brain. As long ago as 2002, the American Academy of Pediatrics announced that any screen time for children under the age of two impedes brain development. Television techniques like cuts, edits, zooms, pans, and sudden noises physically change the young brain.

Every hour of TV that toddlers watch each day, furthermore, increases by ten percent the likelihood that by the age of seven these children will experience attention deficit difficulties. Research shows that television watching by the very young correlates with traits associated with attention deficit hyperactivity disorder.

This information calls in question, surely, the widespread practice in the United States of placing babies sixth months to two years of age in front of TV and computer screens for as long as two hours a day. It also suggests that the seventy percent of young children in the U.S. who have television sets in their bedrooms are not being well served. In fact, Dr. Dina L. G. Borzekowski of John Hopkins headed a study that showed that elementary school children with TV's in their bedrooms consistently scored lower on math, reading, and language arts tests than did children without TV.[23] A French report completed in 2004 found that the more TV children watched, the more unruly they became as they got older.

Relationships in the electronic age

The fascinating products of digital technology tempt us to forget that human beings are a social species and that the development of the human brain depends upon interacting with others. Children learn best from real-life relationships. For instance, when a group of twelve to fifteen-month-olds was shown on television how to use a puppet, they had to watch the TV video six times before they could imitate it. When real people taught them how to use a puppet, they were able to imitate the action immediately. Social interaction sculpts connections among neurons that affect the brain's shape, size, and function.[24]

Unlike adults who hold and talk to children, television and computers neither comfort young children nor teach them how to relate to others. Television screens never give hugs, and they do not teach children where to stand during a conversation, how much eye contact is the right amount, how to gesture, or how to interpret the meanings of facial expressions. From television and computers, children do not learn to understand others or to empathize. Only real contact with adults helps children acquire fundamental social skills such as grasping the emotional meaning of a simple gesture or comprehending another's pain. Every relationship leaves its imprint on the brain. If we lose our social skills, we lose our humanity.[25] Unfortunately, the time children spend with digital media is time that they are not using to develop real-world, real-time, personal relationships.

Furthermore, television, computer, and video screens do not teach young people their native language. Children learn language from conversing with adults face-to-face. In 1900, children talked to adults about seven and a half hours a day. Today children talk to adults about seven minutes a day. In 1945 in the United States, the average number of words in the written vocabulary of a child between the ages of six and fourteen years was twenty-five thousand.

Today in the United States the average number of words in the written vocabulary of six to fourteen-year-olds is ten thousand.

The less children converse with adults, the fewer words they learn. A 2001 study of German children conducted in Mainz, Germany, for instance, showed that twenty percent of all four year olds were given few opportunities to have long talks with adults. As a result, they suffered significant language delays. These children could not understand simple requests, had a very limited grasp of concepts, did not articulate clearly, and knew few words. The sole cause of these disturbing problems, it turned out, was the absence of regular conversations with caring adults. The vocabulary that parents use when they talk to children and the frequency of their conversations matters greatly. The wider and more varied a parent's vocabulary when he or she speaks to a child, the richer the child's vocabulary will be, and thus the higher his IQ. When adults talk regularly and often to children, face-to-face, they help them develop both intellectually and socially.[26]

Love your brain, improve your life, make a difference

This book challenges you to make a difference in your community by designing a brain-friendly environment based on the discoveries of neuroscience. We have noted in this final chapter a few specific features appropriate to a brain-friendly environment. Throughout this book, furthermore, the findings of neuroscience call for the specific actions listed below. These actions can change our communities—our homes, schools, and workplaces—and improve the world. Neuroscience shows us that:

- Hard work and self-discipline can heal the brain and raise IQ. Work with care, mindfulness, and self-discipline.

- Attaching meaning and positive emotions to schoolwork aids the memory. Find meaning; celebrate successes.

- Fear and stress damage body and brain alike. Drive out fear; minimize stress.

- Relationships help determine our intellectual ability, emotional balance and personality traits. Build positive relationships.

- The brain's mirror neurons unite us with others. They let us feel another's emotion and imitate another's action. Imitate only worthy behavior. Do only things that merit emulation.

- Everyone wants to belong. Belonging generates rewarding feelings of pleasure. Help others belong; include everyone.

- Social pain is real. Not belonging triggers pain in two regions of the brain. Never cause any human being social distress.

- Emotion is always with us, expanding our experiences and influencing memory. Although emotion easily dominates the brain, we can use reason to regulate and manage emotion. To manage emotion, learn to think deeply about the thinking process.

- Mindfulness—paying close attention with a receptive mind—helps us find meaning in the moment and see the moment in a new light. Mindfulness is the antithesis of running on automatic pilot. Be mindful.

- Human beings are moral by nature. Judging between right and wrong is an innate ability. Local culture teaches us, however, to denounce as wrong what our culture denounces and applaud as right what our local culture applauds.

Transcend the constraints of culture's narrow code. See with an open mind.

- Changing one's moral position, which is wired into the brain's circuits, is very difficult. Analyze your moral principles. Do they need to be changed?

- Regard the Earth itself and its inhabitants, living and non-living, human and non-human, as equal in value to yourself. Love.

Chapter 6: Endnotes

1. On music and the brain, see Oliver Sacks, *Musicophilia: Tales of Music and the Brain* (New York: Alfred A. Knopf, 2007), pp. xiii, 30-40. See also Daniel J. Levitin, *This is Your Brain on Music* (New York: Plume, 2006), pp. 27; 108-111; 228-236.

2. Levitin, p. 226. See also on the regions affected by music, pp. 208-230; 85-87.

3. Rita Carter, *Mapping the Mind* (Berkeley: University of California Press, 1998), pp. 108-109; Norman Doidge, M.D. *The Brain that Changes Itself* (New York: Viking, 2007), pp., 289-290.

4. Levitin, pp. 226-227; Sacks, pp. 31-32; 38; Peter Perret and Janet Fox. *A Well-Tempered Mind* (Washington D.C.: Dana Press, 2004), pp. 2-3; 12-13; 19-20; 47; 69-77.

5. Music creates social ties. See Karen Schrock, "Why Music Moves Us," *Scientific American Mind* (July/August, 2009), pp. 32-37. Music affects the brain's reward centers, language centers, memory, and creates social bonds. It also transmits knowledge and represents emotional states. It enlists many parts of the brain. See Mary Carmichael, "Sing, Brain, Sing," an interview with Daniel Levitin of McGill University in *Newsweek* (September 22, 2008), p. 56; Melissa Healy, "Making Music is What Fires the Brain," *The Oregonian* (10 Mar. 2010), C1; C4.

6. Jane M. Healy, Ph.D. *Endangered Minds* (New York: Simon & Schuster,1990), pp. 170, 179, 182-183; Jane M. Healy, *Your Child's Growing Mind* (New York: Bantam, Doubleday, 1994), pp. 47-71; "Understanding TV's Effects on the Developing Brain," AAP News Reprint, May 1998. <http://www.aap.org/advocacy.>

7. Gretchen Reynolds, "Phys Ed: Your Brain on Exercise," *The New York Times* (7 July 2010),<http://well.blogs.nytimes.com/2010/07/07>; See also Gretchen Reynolds, "Phys Ed; Can Exercise Make Kids Smarter?" *The New York Times* (15 Sept. 2010). < http://www.blogs.nytimes.com/2010/09/15/phys-ed-can-exercise–make-kids-smarter>.

8. Gretchen Reynolds, "Phys Ed: Can Exercise Make Kids Smarter?"; Sandra Aamodt and Sam Wang "Exercise on the Brain," *New York Times* (8 Nov. 2007).

9. Jane M. Healy, Ph.D. *Endangered Minds,* pp. 168-171; Healy, "Understanding TV's effects on the developing brain," AAP News Reprint, May, 1998.< http://www.aap.org/advocacy>

10. Gretchen Reynolds, "Phys Ed: Can Exercise Make Kids Smarter?"; Gretchen Reynolds, "Lobes of Steel," *The New York Times* (August 19, 2007).

11. John Medina, *Brain Rules* (Seattle: Pear Press, 2008), pp. 21-22; anon. "Move Your Body," in *Your Brain at Work* (New York: Dana Alliance for Brain Initiatives and the Conference Board, 2008), pp. 13-14; Michael S. Sweeney, *Brain: The Complete Mind* (Washington D.C., National Geographic, 2009), p. 187; Sue Halpern, "Forgetting is the New Normal," *Your Brain: A User's Guide* (New York: Time, Inc, 2009), p. 75.

12. Robert Stickgold and Jeffrey M. Ellenbogen, "Quiet! Sleeping Brain at Work," *Scientific American Mind* (August/September, 2008), pp. 23-29. See also Roni Cayn Rabin, "Behavior: Napping Can Prime the Brain for Learning," *The New York Times* (23 Feb. 2010). Stickgold and Rabin both report that sleep strengthens memories.

13. On the teenage brain, see Robert Epstein, "The Myth of the Teen Brain," *Scientific American Mind* (April/May, 2007), pp. 57-63; Robert Epstein, letter to the editor, *Time* (May 7, 2007); Alice Park, "What Makes Teens Tick," *Time,* (May 10, 2004), pp. 57-65; Leslie Sabbagh, "The Teen Brain Hard at Work, No, Really," *Scientific American Mind* (August/

September, 2006), pp. 21-23. Epstein shows that environment influences teenagers' choices, thus increasing or diminishing their potential.

14. On the influence of adult vocabulary on children and on parents' immersion in electronic gadgets to the detriment of children, see Julie Scelfo, "The Risks of Parenting While Plugged In," *The New York Times* (June 9, 2010), <http://www.nytimes.com/2010/06/10/garden/10childtech>.

15. Neuroscientist Susan Greenfield contends that young brains are changed by electronic social networking. Facebook, Twitter, instant messaging, chat rooms and watching TV's fast paced shows all change the personalities, thinking, and abilities of young users. Young people develop short attention spans, seek instant gratification, live for the moment, become more self-centered, cannot concentrate, and reduce their ability to understand others. See David Derbyshire, "Social Websites Harm Children's Brains," *Mail Online,* <http://ww.dailymail.co.uk/news/article> (February 24, 2009).

16. Thomas Clayburn, "Video Game Play Improves Eyesight," *Information Week* (March 30, 2009). <http://www.informationweek.com>.

17. Chris Suellentrop, "Playing With Our Heads: Why Video Games are Making Our Kids Smarter—and More Obedient," *UTNE,* (January/February, 2007), pp. 60-63. Suellentrop argues that the benefits of video games do not justify the liabilities.

18. Chris Suellentrop, p. 63.

19. David Dobbs, "A Revealing Reflection," *Scientific American Mind* (April/May 2006), pp. 22-27. Dobbs notes that "observed violence imitates actual violence" and "imitative violence, if reinforced, may be hard to resist. Imitative violence . . . [is] not subject to control."

20. For information on the effects of violence on the brain see Chris Suellentrop, pp. 60ff; Bruce Perry, M.D., Ph.D., lecture delivered at the "Kid's Brain Conference," Metropolitan State College of Denver (Denver: May 20, 2004); Sandra Blakeslee, "Cells that Read Minds," *The New York Times* (January 10, 2006). David Derbyshire, "Social Websites Harm Children's Brains," *Mail Online* (24 February 2009) <http://www.dailymail.co.uk/news/article; Karen Springen, "Why We Tuned Out" *Newsweek* (11 Nov. 2002), p. 60.

21. Marco Iacoboni, *Mirroring People: The New Science of How We Connect with Others* (New York: Farrar, Straus, and Giroux, 2008), pp. 54-69.

22. Iacoboni, p. 208. [italics mine]

23. "TV in Child's Room Sets Off Academic Alert," *The New York Times* (July 5, 2005).

24. Gary Small, Gigi Vorgan, "Meet Your Brain," *Scientific American Mind* (October/November, 2008), pp. 42-49:

25. Small, Vorgan, "Meet Your Brain," p. 49: From ages 8 to 18, young people experience about 8 hours each day of digital and video sensory stimulation. The brain's neural circuitry responds, causing the brain to evolve. "The neural circuits that control the more traditional learning methods are neglected and gradually diminished. The pathways for human interaction and communication weaken as customary one-on-one people skills atrophy."

26. Norbert Herschkowitz told this story in a lecture presented as part of the OHSU Brain Awareness Series. His point, developed in the book co-authored with his wife, is that language development is a social effort requiring adult participation. See Norbert Herschkowitz and Elinor Chapman Herschkowitz, *A Good Start in Life: Understanding Your Child's Brain and Behavior from Birth to Age 6* (New York: Dana Foundation, 2004), pp. 101-102; 198-199.

APPENDIX:

Ways the Brain Learns Best

Teachers must know each student well to capture that
young person's mind and heart... Students respond when
a matter at hand connects... with something important.

Theodore R. Sizer, Horace's School. (New York: Houghton Mifflin Co., 1992, pp.86-87.

PARENTS EXPECT THEIR CHILDREN TO SUCCEED IN SCHOOL,
and educators dedicate their lives to helping young people learn.
Brain research suggests eight teaching strategies which, when used
together, give all students—those who learn easily and those who
have trouble learning academic material—a solid chance at academic success. The eight strategies and their connection to brain
research are described below.

Eight Teaching and Learning strategies

1. Nurture the individual

Create a nurturing learning environment. Only when students
are encouraged to feel capable, not inept; valuable, not negligible;
secure, not afraid; and appreciated, not inadequate will their brains
develop the emotional balance, intellectual attributes, and personality traits that are essential to academic success. A nurturing classroom provides a necessary foundation for student success.

Brain facts: The brain is a social organ. It needs to interact positively with other brains to complete itself. According to brain research, satisfying relationships cause neurons to form connections that encode feelings of security, self-confidence, competence, generosity, and concern for others. If the brain is denied close and encouraging relationships and assailed with constant negative criticism, it wires itself for insecurity and intellectual failure. Deprivation of positive peer interaction wires the brain for emotional imbalance and personality disorders.

2. Collaborate

When students collaborate, they quickly learn that their way of perceiving is not the only way. In addition to learning to value a classmate's point of view, they acquire social skills such as courtesy and patience. They develop the ability to say, "I have listened to you carefully and have been persuaded by your reasoning. Your logic and evidence are more convincing than mine." They also have occasion to teach one another. From collaborating, students learn that those who work together are more likely to succeed than those who work alone.

Brain facts: The brain needs to interact with other human beings in order to complete itself. Collaborating with peers can not only trigger the reward circuit to deliver feelings of pleasure, but also it can generate brain circuits disposed to transcend selfishness and put others first.

3. Make connections to find meaning

Intent on survival, the human brain constantly searches for meaning. In its search for meaning, the brain checks new information against the knowledge and experience it already possesses. If friends were to ask you, for instance, to join them for five days of bicycling in the Colorado mountains, you could understand the full meaning of this invitation—its implications for you personally—by recalling how you felt that weekend when you biked 200 miles on flat terrain. Recalling that adventure would tell you whether or not to accept the invitation.

Students learn when they see meaning in academic lessons, and they see meaning when they can connect the content of the lesson with the *context* of their daily lives. Meaning is a vital pathway to the long-term memory. When we see meaning in new information, we learn and remember it. Work-based activities, problem-based learning, service learning, discovery projects, and integrated classes are well-known instructional methods that most obviously enable students to find meaning by connecting lessons with the real world.

Brain facts: The environment reaches the brain through the body's five senses. The senses send impulses that cause brain cells (neurons) to connect with one another. When neurons form connections, their nucleus becomes larger, the number and length of dendrites increases, and the number of spines that dendrites produce increases.

The brain's speed and power are thus strengthened. When learning experiences do more than trigger the five senses, when they are also redolent with meaning, the brain is inclined to retain them.

4. Do significant work

Purposeless schoolwork trivializes learning, particularly when it is arbitrarily imposed. School work divorced from the real world seems meaningless. When students connect lessons with significant projects, problems, or issues that affect their class, college, or community, however, they see meaning in academic material. Learning academic material in order to fulfill a purpose that holds meaning inspires students to do their best. When academic work holds significance, students do not ask that mournful question, "Why do we have to learn this?"

Brain facts: Because the brain searches constantly to find meaning, it pays attention to and remembers significant lessons.

5. Engage in active, self-regulated learning

Self-regulated learning puts students in charge of their academic success. It asks them to use their minds and bodies as they engage in concrete activities that involve the five senses. To reach academic goals, self-regulated learners design their own projects, search out information leading to independent conclusions, choose, order, organize, investigate, question, and decide. They take the initiative, develop plans, and draw on their particular strengths as they confer with others and investigate sites.

Brain facts: Brain research suggests that self-regulated learning activities help us learn and remember because such activities stimulate the fives senses. Each of the five senses sends information to a particular region of the brain, causing neurons to form circuits in that region. Located in different regions throughout the brain, these circuits provide many hooks, or associations, that facilitate acquiring and recalling new information.

Self-regulated learning also gives the brain time to consolidate and retain new information. Taking time to learn—that is, figuring things out, thinking through problems to find solutions, weighing alternatives, making comparisons, covering less but covering it thoroughly—allows the brain to store information in its long-term memory. Relaxing after a concentrated period of hard work also aids memory.

6. Emphasize critical and creative thinking

Critical thinking is open-minded thinking aimed at achieving the fullest understanding possible. It involves looking systematically at the thought processes that support beliefs, ideas, knowledge, and convictions. To break the hold of emotion and distorted logic, critical thinkers ask specific questions about the subject at issue, scrutinize their own biases, seek solid reasons that support a position, scrutinize evidence to make sure it is reliable, test assumptions and concepts, and consider that conclusions may have unanticipated consequences.

Creative thinkers, on the other hand, generate new, uncommon, unexpected, imaginative insights. Creative thinkers see the familiar from a new perspective, generate fresh solutions to old problems, and change existing inventions. They also invent entirely new theories and things. Everyone is creative. Students use their creativity when they ask questions, contribute to class discussions, or devise a different way to do something. A classroom that encourages creative thinking respects the individual, values integrity and courage, is receptive to all ideas, welcomes questions, has a high tolerance for strangeness, and encourages perseverance.

Brain facts: Located in the frontal cortex is the capacity to reason in an organized way. Reason enables us to do such things as manage emotions, postpone gratification, and exercise sound judgment. The qualities identified with a cultivated "self" are nurtured by reason.

The urge to create arises in part, evidently, from the brain's amazing plasticity. The brain can rewire itself perpetually—can create new patterns perpetually—in response to impulses that reach it from the outside world.

7. Reach high standards

It is the proper aim of all faculty, from elementary school through university, to help students attain high standards. This aim is achieved by teaching in ways that take advantage of the brain's capacity to increase in IQ.

Brain facts: Brain research suggests that it is invariably a mistake to underestimate people. IQ is multiple, not single. It is malleable and learnable, not fixed. Since everyone is intelligent in many ways, and since intelligence can be raised by as much as twenty points, it follows that all students should be encouraged to aim high.

8. Authentic Assessment

Authentic assessment asks students to apply new information about a subject to a real situation for an actual purpose. Composing authentic assessment tasks involves asking, for example: "How do people actually use mathematics? What forms does writing take not just in school and college, but also in practical affairs?" Authentic assessment invites students to apply their knowledge. In addition to authentic assessment, student self-assessment and frequent classroom feedback increase academic success.

Brain facts: The brain has the unique ability to see its mistakes and to correct itself. Regular and timely feedback and the experiences provided by authentic assessment help the brain appraise its own behavior and correct any shortcomings. Authentic assessment also provides a real context for school work. It joins learning with life.

REFERENCES

Aamodt, Sandra and Sam Wang. "Exercise on the Brain." *New York Times*. 8 Nov. 2007. <http://www.nytimes.com/2007/11/08/opinion/08aamodt. html?_r=1>

Beauregard, Mario and Denyse O'Leary. *The Spiritual Brain: A Neuroscientist's Case for the Existence of the Soul*. New York: Harper One, 2007.

Begley, Sharon. "Heard Any Good Stories Lately?" *Newsweek* 22 Sept. 2008: 42.

_____. How the Brain Rewires Itself." *Time*, 29 Jan. 2007: 68-74.

_____. *Train Your Mind, Change Your Brain: How a New Science Reveals Our Extraordinary Potential to Transform Ourselves*. New York: Ballantine Books, 2007.

Blakeslee, Sandra. "Cells that Read Minds." *New York Times* 10 Jan. 2006. <http://www.nytimes.com>

Bloom, Paul. "The Moral Life of Babies." *New York Times*. 3 May, 2010: 2-5. <http://www.nytimes.com/2010/05/09/magazine/09babies>

Brizendine, Louann. *The Female Brain*. New York: Broadway Books, 2006.

Butler, Kiera. "Works Well With Others." *Mother Jones*. Jan./ Feb. 2008: 66-69.

Calvin, William H. *How Brains Think: Evolving Intelligence Then and Now*. New York: Basic Books, 1996.

Campbell, Neil A., Lawrence G. Mitchell, Jane B. Reece. *Biology: Concepts and Connections*. New York: Benjamin Cummings, 1994.

Cacioppo, John T. and William Patrick. *Loneliness: Human Nature and the Need for Social Connection*. New York: W. W. Norton, 2008.

Cardoso, Silvia Helena. "Hardwired for Happiness." The Dana Foundation: 15 Dec. 2006. <http://www.dana.org/printerfriendly.aspx.id=5514>.

Carey, Benedict. "How Nonsense Sharpens the Intellect." *New York Times*, 6 Oct. 2009. <http://www.nytimes.com/2009/10/06.>

Carr, Nicholas. *The Shallows: What the Internet is Doing to Our Brains.* New York: W.W. Norton, 2010.

Carter, Rita. *Mapping the Mind.* Berkeley: University of California Press, 1998.

Carter, Rita, Susan Aldridge, Martyn Page, and Steve Parker. *The Human Brain Book.* London: DK, 2009.

Clayburn, Thomas. "Video Game Play Improves Eyesight." *Information Week.* 30 March, 2009. <http://www.informationweek.com> obb Jr, John B. "Capital." Jan. 2009. A paper written to be delivered at a conference held in Suzhou, China, Jan. 2009.

Cozolino, Louis. *The Neuroscience of Human Relationships: Attachment and the Developing Social Brain.* New York: W. W. Norton, 2006.

Currier, Ken. "Why Are Bad Habits so Hard to Break?" 27 May 2008. *Stuff Your Brain Likes.* <http://www.stuffyourbrainlikes.com>

Damasio, Antonio. *Descartes' Error: Emotion, Reason, and the Human Brain* (New York: Avon Books, 1994.

Davis, Joel. *Mapping the Mind: The Secrets of the Human Brain and How It Works.* Secaucus, NY: Birch Lane, 1997.

Derbyshire, David. "Social Websites Harm Children's Brains." *Mail Online.* 24 Feb. 2009. <http://www.dailymail.co.uk/news/article>

Diamond, Marian and Janet Hopson. *Magic Trees of the Mind: How to Nurture Your Child's Intelligence, Creativity, and Healthy Emotions from Birth Through Adolescence.* New York: Plume Book, 1999.

Dobbs, David. "A Revealing Reflection." *Scientific American Mind.* April/May 2006: 22-27.

Doidge, Norman. *The Brain that Changes Itself: Stories of Personal Triumph from the Frontiers of Brain Science.* New York: Viking, 2007.

Edelman, Gerald. *Second Nature: Brain Science and Human Knowledge.* New Haven: Yale University Press.

Eisenberger, Naomi and Matthew Lieberman, with K.D. Williams. "Does Rejection Hurt? An fMRI Study of Social Exclusion." *Science.* vol. 302. No. 5643. October 2003: 290-292.

Eisenberger, Naomi and Matthew Lieberman. "The Pains and Pleasures of Social Life." *Science.* vol 323. No. 5916. February 2009: 890-891.

_____. "Why it Hurts to be Left Out: The Neurocognitive Overlap between Physical and Social Pain." *Trends in Cognitive Sciences.*2004: 8, 294-300.

Elkhonon Goldberg. *The Executive Brain: Frontal Lobes and the Civilized Mind.* Oxford: Oxford University Press, 2001.

Epstein, Robert. "The Myth of the Teen Brain." *Scientific American Mind.* April/ May 2007: 57-63.

_____. Letter. *Time.* 7 May 2007.

Fleischman, John. *Phineas Gage: A Gruesome but True Story about Brain Science.* Boston: Houghton Mifflin, 2002.

Gardner, Howard. *Five Minds for the Future.* Boston: Harvard Business Press, 2008.

_____. *Frames of Mind: The Theory of Multiple Intelligences.* New York: Basic Books, 1983.

Gazzaniga, Michael. *The Ethical Brain.* New York: Dana Press, 2005.

_____. *Human: The Science Behind What Makes Us Unique.* New York: Harper Collins, 2008.

Gill, Victoria. "Singing 'rewires' Damaged Brain." *BBC News.* <http://news.bbc. co.uk/2/hi/8526699.stm>

Goleman, Daniel. *Emotional Intelligence.* New York: Bantam Books, 1995.

_____, Richard Boyatzis. "Social Intelligence and the Biology of Leadership." *Harvard Business Review.* Sept. 2008: 74-81.

_____. *Social Intelligence: The New Science of Human Relationships.* New York: Bantam Books. 2007.

Greenfield, Susan A. *The Human Brain: A Guided Tour.* New York: Basic Books, 1997.

Greybiel, Ann. OHSU Brain Awareness Lecture Series. OMSI. Portland, Oregon, 23 Oct. 2002.

Gudrais, Elizabeth. "The Developing Child." *Harvard Magazine.* April, 2009: 34-81.

Gunnar, Megan. "The Impact of Early Adversity on Brain Development: How the Brain Recovers from Stress." Lecture at Oregon Conference on Early Childhood. Portland, Oregon. 1 May 2009.

Halpern, Sue. "Forgetting is the New Normal." *Your Brain: A User's Guide.* Ed. Jeffrey Kluger. New York: *Time,* 2009. 72-76.

Healy, Jane M. *Endangered Minds: Why Children Don't Think and What We Can Do About It.* New York: Simon & Schuster, 1990.

_____. *Your Child's Growing Mind: A Beginner's Guide to Learning and Brain Development from Birth to Adolescence.* rev. ed. New York: Doubleday, 1994.

_____. "Understanding TV's Effect on the Developing Brain." AAP News Reprint, May 1998. <http://www.aap.org/advocacy>

Healy, Melissa. "Making Music is What Fires the Brain." *The Oregonian.* 10 March 2010: C1; C4.

Herschkowitz, Norbert and Elinore Chapman Herschkowitz. *A Good Start in Life: Understanding Your Child's Brain and Behavior from Birth to Age 6.* 2nd ed. New York: Dana Press, 2004.

Hyman, Steven. "Susceptibility and 'Second Hits.'" *States of Mind: New Discoveries about How Our Brains Make Us Who We Are.* Ed. Roberta Conlan. New York: The Dana Press and John Wiley & Sons, 1999. 9-28.

Iacoboni, Marco. *Mirroring People: The New Science of How We Connect with Others.* New York: Farrar, Straus, and Giroux, 2008.

Interlandi, Janeen, "Mysteries of Memory: New Research Explores How the Brain Records and then Recalls Events" *Newsweek.* 22 Sept. 2008. <http://www.newsweek.com/2008/09/12mysteries-lof-memory.html>

Johnson, Elaine. *Contextual Teaching and Learning: What It Is and Why It's Here to Stay.* Thousand Oaks, CA: Corwin, 2002.

_____. "Changing Our Systems By Changing Our Brains: The Leverage in Mindfulness." *The Systems Thinker.* Vol. 21. No. 7, Sept. 2010: 2-6.

Johnson, Samuel. *The Idler,* no. 44. 17 Feb., 1759.

Kagan, Jerome. *An Argument for Mind.* New Haven: Yale University Press, 2006.

Kluger, Jeffery. "Language and the Baby Brain." *Your Brain: A User's Guide.* Ed. Jeffrey Kluger. New York: Time, 2009. 26-30.

_____. "What Makes Us Moral?" *Time* 3 Dec. 2007: 54-60.

_____. "What Makes Us Moral?" *Your Brain: A User's Guide.* New York: Time, 2009. 84-89.

Lambert, Kelley. "Depressingly Easy." *Scientific American Mind.* Aug/Sept. 2008:35-35.

Langer, Ellen. J. *The Power of Mindful Learning.* Cambridge: Perseus Books, 1997.

LeDoux, Joseph. *The Emotional Brain: The Mysterious Underpinnings of Emotional Life*. New York: Simon & Schuster, 1996.

_____. "The Power of Emotions." *States of Mind: New Discoveries about How Our Brains Make Us Who We Are*. Ed. Roberta Conlan. New York: The Dana Press and John Wiley & Sons, 1999. 123-149.

_____. *Synaptic Self: How Our Brains Become Who We Are*. New York: Viking, 2002.

Lehrer, Johan. "How We Decide: From Brains to Behavior." OHSU Brain Awareness Lecture Series. Newmark Theater, Portland, Oregon. 1 Feb. 2010.

Lieberman, Matthew D. "Social Cognitive Neuroscience." *Encyclopedia of Social Psychology*. Eds. R. F. Baumeister and K. D. Vohs. Thousand Oaks: Sage, 2007.

Lieberman, Matthew D. and Naomi I. Eisenberger. "Pains and Pleasures of Social Life." *Science*. vol. 323. 13 Feb. 2009: 890-891. <http://www.sciencemag.org.> downloaded Aug. 2010.

Leitzel, Katherine. "The Other Brain Cells." *Scientific American Mind*. June/July, 2008: 7.

Lemonick, Michael. "The Many Flavors of Memory." *Your Brain: A User's Guide*. Ed. Jeffrey Kluger. New York: Time, 2009. 78-81.

Levitin, Daniel. "Sing, Brain, Sing." Interview by Mary Carmichael. *Newsweek*. 22 Sept. 2008: 56.

Levitin, Daniel J. *This is Your Brain on Music: The Science of a Human Obsession*. New York: Plume, 2007.

Lewis, Thomas, Fari Amini, and Richard Lannon. *A General Theory of Love*. New York: Vintage Books, 2000.

Marmot, Michael. *The Status Syndrome: How Social Standing Affects Our Health and Longevity*. New York: Henry Holt, 2004.

Maturana, Humberto and Pille Bunnell. "The Biology of Business: Love Expands Intelligence." *Reflections*. Vol 1, no. 2: 10-12.

_____. "Biosphere, Homosphere, and Robosphere: What Has That to Do with Business?" Paper based on Maturana's lecture at a meeting of the Society for Organizational Learning. Amherst, Mass. June, 1998. <http://www.sol-ne.org/res/wp/maturana> downloaded 27 Jan. 1999.

McEwen, Bruce. "Stress and the Brain." *States of Mind: New Discoveries about How Our Brains Make Us Who We Are.* Ed. Roberta Conlan. New York: The Dana Press and John Wiley Sons, 1999. 81-101.

Meadows, Donella. "Voice of a Global Citizen." 5 July 2008 <http://www.sustainabilityinstitute.org/DHM_archive/index> Downloaded Aug. 2009.

Medina, John. *Brain Rules: 12 Principles for Surviving and Thriving at Work, Home, and School.* Seattle: Pear, 2008.

Merzenich, Michael. "Neuroplasticity: The Amazing Adaptability of the Brain." OHSU Brain Awareness Lecture Series. Newmark Theater, Portland, Oregon. 26 Jan. 2010.

Meyer, Jerrold S. and Linda F. Quenzer. *Psychopharmacology: Drugs, the Brain and Behavior.* Sunderland, Mass: Sinazier Assoc, 2005.

Moll, Jorge and Ricardo de Oliveira-Souza. "When Morality is Hard to Like: How do We Juggle Evidence and Emotions to Make a Moral Decision?" *Scientific American Mind.* Feb./Mar. 2008: 30-35.

"Move Your Body." *Your Brain at Work.* New York: Dana Alliance for Brain Initiatives and the Conference Board, 2008:13-14.

Myers, David G. "The Powers and Perils of Intuition: Understanding the Nature of Our Gut Instincts." *Scientific American Mind.* June/July, 2007: 24-29.

Nash, Madeline. "The Gift of Mimicry: Why Monkeys See and Do, Why Babies Smile at Mothers, and Why Our Skin Crawls at Scary Movies." *Time* 29 Jan. 2007: 109-111.

Nass, Clifford, Eyal Ophir, and Anthony Wagner. Their research on multitasking discussed in *Computer World.* 1 September 2009 <http://www.computerworld.com>

National Institute of Neurological Disorders and Strokes (NINDS) <Ninds.nih.gov/disorders/brain_basics/know_your_brain.htm>

Neville, Helen. "Effects of Environment on the Brain." Lecture at Oregon Conference on Early Childhood. Portland, Oregon. 1 May 2009.

Nisbett, Richard E. *Intelligence and How to Get It.* New York: W.W. Norton, 2009.

Norden, Jeanette. *Understanding the Brain.* Chantilly, VA: The Teaching Company, 2007.

_____. Lecturer. "Understanding the Brain." DVD. The Teaching Company, 2007.

Oliwenstein, Lori. "The Most Important Sex Organ." *Your Brain: A User's Guide.* Ed. Jeffrey Kluger. New York: *Time,* 2009. 33-36.

Oxford English Dictionary. Compact edition. OUP, 1971.

Park, Alice. "What Makes Teens Tick." *Time.* 10 May 2004: 57-65.

Perret, Peter and Janet Fox. *A Well-Tempered Mind: Using Music to Help Children Listen and Learn.* Dana Press: New York, 2004.

Pinel, John P. J., with Maggie Edwards. *A Colorful Introduction to the Anatomy of the Human Brain: A Brain and Psychology Coloring Book.* Boston: Allyn and Bacon, 1998.

Pinker, Steven. "The Moral Instinct." *New York Times Magazine* 13 Jan. 2009. <http://www.nytimes.com/2008/01/13/magazine/13Psychology-t.html>

Rabin, Roni Cayn. "Behavior: Napping Can Prime the Brain for Learning." *New York Times.* 23 Feb. 2010. <http://www.nytimes.com/2010/02/23/health/research/23beha.? >

Ramachandran, Vilayanur S. and Diane Rogers-Ramachandran, "I See, But I Don't Know," *Scientific American Mind.* Dec. 2008/ Jan. 2009: 20-22.

Ratey, John. *A User's Guide to the Brain: Perception, Attention, and the Four Theaters of the Brain.* New York: Vintage, 2002.

Restak, Richard. *The Secret Life of the Brain.* New York: The Dana Press and Joseph Henry Press, 2001.

Rettner, Rachael. "Multitasking Only Lets You Use Half a Brain." MSNBC.com <http://www.msnbc.msn.com/id/36582695/ns/health-behavior>

Reynolds, Gretchen. "Lobes of Steel." *New York Times.* 19 August 2007. <http://www.nytimes.com/2007/08/19/sports/playmagazine/0819play-brain.html?>

――――――――――. "Phys Ed: Can Exercise Make Kids Smarter?" *New York Times.* 15 Sept. 2010. <http://www.blogs.nytimes.com/2010/09/15/phys-ed-can-exercise-make-kids-smarter/>

――――――――――. "Phys Ed: Your Brain on Exercise." *New York Times.* 7 July 2010. <http://www.well.blogs.nytimes.com/20210/07/07

Richtel, Matt. "Hooked on Gadgets, and Paying a Mental Price." *New York Times* 6 June 2010. <http://www.nytimes.com/2010/06/07>, downloaded 10 June 2010.

Rizzolatti, Giacomo, Leonardo Fogassi, Vittorio Gallese. "Mirrors in the Mind." *Scientific American.* Nov. 2006: 54-69.

Rock, David. "Managing with the Brain in Mind." *Strategy+Business*. Autumn, 2009. Issue 56: 59-65.

Rock, David and Jeffrey Schwartz. "The Neuroscience of Leadership." *Strategy+Business*. Summer 2006. Issue 43: 2-10.

Christine Rosen. "The Myth of Multitasking." *New Atlantis: A Journal of Technology & Society*. No. 20. Spring, 2008, pp. 105-110. <www. thenewatlantis.com>

Rosen, Jeffrey. "The Brain on the Stand." *New York Times Magazine*, 11 March, 2007: <http://www.nytimes.com/preview20>

Sabbagh, Leslie. "The Teen Brain Hard at Work, No, Really." *Scientific American Mind*. Aug./ Sept. 2006: 21-23.

Sacks, Oliver. *Musicophilia: Tales of Music and the Brain*. New York: Alfred A. Knopf, 2007.

Sapolsky, Robert M. *Biology and Human Behavior: The Neurological Origins of Individuality*, 2nd ed. Chantilly, VA: The Teaching Company, 2005.

_____. Lecturer. "Biology and Human Behavior: The Neurological Origins of Individuality." DVD. The Teaching Company, 2005.

_____. OHSU Brain Awareness Series. OMSI. Portland, Oregon. 5 Feb. 2003.

_____. *Why Zebras Don't Get Ulcers: An Updated Guide to Stress, Stress-Related Disease, and Coping*. New York: W. H. Freeman, 1994.

Scelfo, Julie. "The Risks of Parenting While Plugged In." *New York Times*. 9 June 2010. http://www.nytimes.com/2010/06/10/garden/10childtech

Schacter, Daniel L. *Searching for Memory: The Brain, the Mind, and the Past*. New York: Basic Books, 1996.

Scharmer, C. Otto. *Theory U: Leading from the Future As It Emerges*. San Francisco: Berrett-Koehler, 2009.

Schrock, Karen. "Why Music Moves Us." *Scientific American Mind*. July/Aug 2009: 32-37.

Schwartz, Jeffrey M. and Sharon Begley. *The Mind and the Brain: Neuroplasticity and the Power of Mental Force*. New York: Regan Books, 2002.

Senge, Peter. "Foreword." *Theory U: Leading from the Future As It Emerges*. By C. Otto Scharmer. San Francisco: Berrett-Koehler, 2009.

Siegel, Daniel J. *The Developing Mind: Toward a Neurobiology of Interpersonal Experience*. New York: The Guilford Press, 1999.

_____. *The Mindful Brain: Reflection and Attunement in the Cultivation of Well-Being*. New York: W. W. Norton, 2007.

Shermer, Michael. "Don't Be Evil: Enron, Google and the Evolutionary Psychology of Corporate Environment." *Scientific American Mind*. Feb./ March 2008: 58-65.

Small, Gary and Gigi Vorgan. "Meet Your Brain." *Scientific American Mind*. July/ Aug. 2008: 42-49.

Sousa, David A. *How the Brain Learns: A Classroom Teacher's Guide*. Reston, VA: NASSP, 1995.

Springen, Karen. "Why We Tuned Out." *Newsweek*. 11 Nov. 2002: 60.

Sternberg, Esther M. *The Balance Within: The Science Connecting Health and Emotions*. New York: W. H. Freeman, 2001.

Sternberg, Robert J. *Successful Intelligence: How Practical and Creative Intelligence Determine Success in Life*. New York: Plume Book, 1997.

Stickgold, Robert and Jeffrey M. Ellenbogen. "Quiet! Sleeping Brain at Work." *Scientific American Mind*. Aug./ Sept. 2008: 23-29.

Suellentrop, Chris. "Playing with Our Heads: Why Video Games are Making Our Kids Smarter—and More Obedient." *UTNE* Jan./ Feb. 2007:60-63.

Sweeney, Michael S. *Brain: The Complete Mind*. Washington, D.C.: National Geographic, 2009.

Swimme, Brian and Thomas Berry. *The Universe Story: from the Primordial Flaring Forth to the Ecozoic Era—A Celebration of the Unfolding of the Cosmos*. San Francisco: Harper Collins, 1992.

Sylwester, Robert. *A Celebration of Neurons: An Educator's Guide to the Human Brain*. Alexandria, VA. Association for Supervision and Curriculum Development, 1995.

Szalavitz, Maia. "Kindness 1012." *Time*. 24 May 2010: 46.

"TV in Child's Room Sets Off Academic Alert." *New York Times*. 5 July 2005.

Wallis, Claudia. "Gen M: The Multitasking Generation." *Time* 27 March 2006: 48-58.

Westerhoff, Nikolas. "Set in Our Ways." *Scientific American Mind*. Dec./Jan 2009: 44-49.

Widerman, Michael. "Why It's So Hard to Be Happy." *Scientific American Mind*. Feb./Mar 2007: 36-43.

Wright, Robert. "How We Make Life-and-Death Decisions." *Time*. 29 Jan. 2007: 116.

Zogby International. "Results of the 2010 WBI [Workplace Bullying Institute] U. S. Workplace Bullying Survey." <http:///www.workplacebullying.org/research/WBI-NatlSurvey2010.html>

Zogby International and Workplace Bullying Institute (WBI). "Results of the 2007 WBI U. S. Workplace Bullying Survey. <http://www.workplacebullying.org/research/WBI-Zogby2007Survey.html>

INDEX